Anxiety Warrior

VOLUME TWO

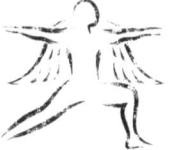

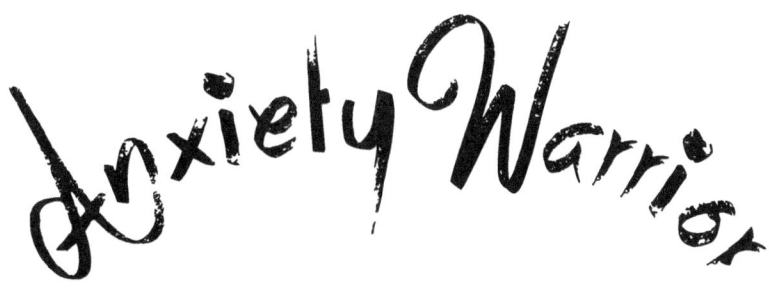

Anxiety Warrior

VOLUME TWO

More great tools for your journey to emotional freedom

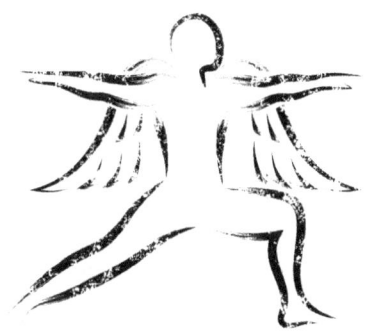

ELKE SCHOLZ

WITH CONTRIBUTORS

The Artist's Reply

Published by The Artist's Reply
Bracebridge, Ontario, Canada

ISBN 978-1-989214-06-0 (pbk.)
ISBN 978-1-989214-05-3 (ePub))

Cover art, design, typesetting:
Magdalene Carson, New Leaf Publication Design

This book is written in Canadian English.

PERMISSIONS
Every attempt has been made to locate the sources of photographs
and other visuals. Should there be errors or omissions, please
contact the author for correction in future printings.

DISCLAIMER
The author and contributors of this book do not dispense medical
advice or prescribe the use of any technique as a form of treatment
for physical, emotional, mental or medical problems without the
advice of a physician, either directly or indirectly. The intent of the
author and contributors is to offer only information of a general
nature to help you in your exploration for spiritual and emotional
well-being. In the event you use any of this information for yourself
or others, the publisher, author, and contributors assume no
responsibility for your actions. The publisher does not endorse,
nor is responsible for, the contributors and their contributions.

To all of us who stumble on anxiety,
we are all Chikara Warriors.
We can do this!

Contents

Acknowledgements   xi

Introduction   1

How to Use This Book   7

What Is Anxiety?   9

What Is Anxiety?   11
1. Generalized Anxiety Disorder (GAD)   16
2. Social Phobia   17
3. Panic Disorder   18
4. Agoraphobia   20
5. Phobias   21
6. Post Traumatic Stress Disorder (PTSD)   22
7. Obsessive Compulsive Disorder (OCD)   23

Eleven Layers of Anxiety   26
1. Substances   26
2. Physiological   28
3. Reality   28
4. Overstimulation   30
5. Cultural and social beliefs   31
6. Self-doubt   33
7. Perfectionism   33
8. Negative thinking   33
9. High sensitivity   34
10. Memories   35
11. Traumas   35

Empowering Your Anxiety Warrior 37

Authenticity: Is It Something We Really Want?
Elke Scholz 39

Anxiety and the Body
Dr. Nick Bianchi 49

Anxiety Meets Compassion
Nicki Koethner 57

A Naturopathic Medical Approach to Treating
Anxiety
Dr. Colette Harman 64

Tea and Stress
Craig Denstadt 75

Yerba Maté: The Healthy Energizer Brought to You
by Nature's Synergy
Rosscoe Marks 84

Essential Oils for Anxiety
Chantelle Denstedt 92

The Sacred Tree
Susan O'Connell 104

Yoga and Anxiety
Angie Davis 121

Managing Anxiety and Stress with Kundalini Yoga
Susan Allen — Sat Akal Kaur 139

The Radiant Fire: Confronting the Critic and
Nurturing the Inner Child
Krystal Demaine 151

Managing Anxiety with Breathing
Dr. Colette Harman 163

Guided Imagery: How Your Mind Can Help You
Reduce Pain and Cope Better with Stress
Dr. Roxanne Daleo 172

Boundaries
Elke Scholz 180

Transitional Poetry 187

Transitional Poetry 188

The peace and quiet of DEAD
Elke Scholz 189

Take this pill
Reilly Scott 191

What is courage?
Elke Scholz 193

Life waiting for You
Emma Scholz Bertrand 195

Soul Destiny
Elke Scholz 196

Chikara Warrior Stories 197

Chikara Warrior Stories and Senjutsu 198

A Different Kind of Warrior Now
Kathryn Boland 199

Anxiety Can Lead You Further
Barb Campbell 206

The Miracle of Pets
Sarah Clifford 209

Work Anxiety
Magdalene Carson 214

A Moment Can Change a Life
Angie Davis 218

I'll Be Fine
Amanda Duncan 224

A Couple's Experience: His and Her Viewpoints
Amanda and Noel Duncan 230

When Anxiety Encounters Traditional
Chinese Medicine
Kory Sadie Ford 239

The Masks We Wear
Karen Girard 244

House of Cards to Happiness
Tracey Howarth   *252*

Pushing Through My Diagnosis
Meaghan O'Neill   *258*

I Got This: Unlocking Your Instincts
Nancy Osborne   *261*

A Caregiver's Chronicle
M. Secord   *269*

Seeing Past the Noise
Melanie Walbridge   *277*

Senjutsu of Chikara Warriors   *281*

Senjutsu (tactics) of the Chikara Warrior Stories   *283*

A Mental Checklist   *286*

Supportive Charts   *288*

Empowering Your Own Anxiety Warrior   *291*

Glossary   *295*

References   *301*

About the Contributors   *305*

About the Author   *317*

Acknowledgements

First, I would like to thank my children, Alec and Emma. They may not always understand me and my anxiety, however, they love me all the same. They are my most important achievement. Writing a book on anxiety has itself been a source of anxiety for me, and we have found some humour in that!

And I thank my good family doctor, Dr. Allison Small, who took the time to get to know me. She waited and she trusted me to come to her when I needed to, for she saw the anxiety in me before I saw it myself. As a medical doctor she is aware of self-care and has always been respectful, open to healing, being thorough, listening to me and supporting me.

To my dear colleagues and professionals who inspire me, I am grateful for the network of mutual support and encouragement we have created. While we may not see each other often, we are always available and in touch, which is sustaining and motivating.

I am also grateful to my friends and community for all their assistance, sponsorship, encouragement, and enthusiasm in this book and *The Anxiety Warrior Project: Celebrating Living Life Well, a symposium,* where this book was officially launched. Both the book and the project have been a collective effort and certainly not a solitary journey.

Thank you Scott Williams, a wonderful editor, I hope you always have time for me. We have put in many years and hours together. You are gracious and have a gift of being in the reader's chair.

Thank you, Susanne Mika, my assistant, for believing in me and the work.

To Magdalene Carson, for listening and chatting with me, not always about designing, for letting me cry and laugh. For all the collaborative fun we have when we are on fire about designing! For being Exalted Warriors together!

Thank you, Ted Lute, for fresh eyes at the final hour for a read, a friendly critique, and for the Japanese Anime word exploration. You are an avid reader and happily said "Yes!"

Thank you to all the contributors. You are so passionate about your work and about empowering people. Your sharing and stories fill my heart over and over again. Your encouragement and belief in the good works, give hope.

And to all of you around the world, who believe in me and the work. People have asked me where I get the energy. Your letters, emails, personal stories, and triumphs go right to my heart and fuel my fire.

Introduction

Are you reading this book because anxiety has become a constant companion? Is it with you everywhere, all the time? Or hits you unexpectedly? Does it feel like the worst feeling ever? Do you feel like a victim losing? Or like an empowered warrior? When you feel anxiety, it feels like you are fighting it. Yet somehow anxiety can be a gift, an opportunity. A battle that does not have violent casualties; instead, these casualties are the many layers of anxiety. The battle then is to overcome and to manage these many layers of anxiety.

In the first volume of *Anxiety Warrior*, I share what I have learned from years of research and practice about managing anxiety. Included are five writers; speakers, teachers, and facilitators who offer unique insights and perspectives. They are passionate about their topics and live them.

As I was about to launch and celebrate *Anxiety Warrior* and "The Anxiety Warrior Project: learning symposium of celebrating life and lowering anxiety," I realized how many community resources are available to us, and included some of them.

In developing *Anxiety Warrior Volume Two* and a second symposium, I continue to be in awe of what I am learning and of the resources that can help people manage anxiety and thrive. The two volumes together make a complete resource for managing and lowering anxiety. Each has a rich uniqueness in its offering.

Here in this edition are chapters on the benefits of teas, essential oils, yoga, Chinese medicine, nature, expressive arts, music therapy, breath work, nutritional health, aging and planning, and mental challenges, all by people passionate about their work and lives. You will notice that some themes are common and overlap, which shows their strength and success. Also included are personal stories about overcoming challenging life situations, contributed by people I consider heroes for what they've accomplished. All the contributors are Chikara warriors. "Chikara" is a Japanese word meaning power, strength, and capability, and suggests discipline and honour. I had been looking for a word to describe an anxiety warrior as a hero, and one who is more than just a warrior.

I know from my own personal and professional experience that we *can* lower our levels of anxiety and that it takes determination and courage.

Today I manage my anxiety.

I have had challenges with anxiety all my life, but I did not always know it. As a child I had migraines, tummy aches, and flu-ish feelings so often that I had to miss school. My mom believed my symptoms, but my dad did not think that I was truly sick. Often I would be sick before a test or presentation. I also would cry easily in class if teachers raised their voices, even when I was not the target. I remember as a teen feeling angry, useless, hopeless, misunderstood, and very alone, until I met two very special teachers, Mrs. Yeo, my Creative English teacher, and Mr. Hodwitz, my Drama teacher. They saved my life. After their classes I felt I could be okay in the world.

In my 20s, at times I would feel "out of myself." At the time, I could not recall how or why it came on. An urgent feeling would hijack me and I felt a need to run away, usually to a nearby meadow. I felt I had to hide. Sometimes, I would run along the beach and curl up in a fetal position beside a dune until the feeling subsided and I felt safe and could breathe normally again. At that time I thought I was "crazy." It was my secret. As I write here, it is the first time I have ever told anyone this. I know now that it was trauma and anxiety related. That is another story.

Twenty years ago I went through periods when I had trouble getting out of bed. I would send my son off to school and then go back to bed until he came home. Sometimes I would get dressed, sometimes not. When out of bed, I would sit and stare at my work or sit outside and stare. I had no idea that I might be anxious or depressed. I felt immobilized and had no idea about how to get out and be different. I denigrated myself. I had gone to see one counsellor and she said I was "my own worst enemy." I really did not know what she meant by that, and I was too vulnerable to risk asking. That comment only made me feel worse. Looking back, I see that she did not give me strategies or direction so that I could learn how to be my own best friend.

Fifteen years ago, I didn't sleep for two years. I would not fight it and instead would lie awake and rest as best I could, so I could work and carry on. Friends encouraged me to go to the doctor because I could get very sick. One day, I decided to go for a spa weekend of Turkish sauna, hot tub, and massage. But despite the spa treatment, my body remained exhausted. I could barely walk and get ready for bed, yet I stared awake at the ceiling all night. I knew then that I needed to see my doctor. In tears I told her that I could not sleep and wondered if I had anxiety? She said yes, and that she had been waiting for me to come to her.

My good doctor would not give me sleeping pills unless I promised her that I would go to therapy. I was affronted, as I didn't think that I needed therapy. However, I agreed since I needed so badly to sleep. This began a journey of discovery that shaped my personal and professional life.

I remember some key points of change and awareness.

+ Twenty-one years ago, I drove my silver Ford station wagon to a workshop. It was a fine sunny day, traffic was good and I felt good. About 20 minutes later, I felt sad and my mood dropped. I felt sick. Nothing had changed except that I was further down the highway. I noticed this, changed channels in my mind and thought of a fun, happy fantasy. At the time I did not fully realize what I had done.

+ Just over twelve years ago, I remember very clearly driving in my van down Manitoba Street in Bracebridge, on another sunny day, thinking *I have all my fingers and toes, I can see, hear, I have a lovely home, I am able, healthy, and have two great kids, so why am I not dancing in the streets celebrating?* Instead, I felt horrible. I was determined to change.

Have you ever met those people who, when you ask how they are, say "SUPER! GREAT!" And they mean it. I wanted to be one of those people.

I was determined to change channels. And so, I began this journey of discovery.

I'm sharing my personal and professional experiences with you because every week half a million Canadians will miss work due to stress/anxiety.[1] About 30 percent of girls and 20 percent of boys have had an anxiety disorder, according to data from the U.S. National Institute of Mental Health,[2] and most people who come to my private clinic suffer from anxiety. The success that my clients have achieved and the positive response to my talks on anxiety have fuelled my passion about lowering levels of anxiety in a way that is approachable, easy, and accessible for everyone who needs it.

Can you imagine a life without anxiety? Is it reasonable to think one could not ever have anxiety again? That is not likely. Anxiety is part of the human spectrum of feelings. Anxiety can be a gift or a clue, notifying us that we need to pay attention to something, that perhaps something is amiss. However, we can have a life where anxiety does not control our lives, our decisions, and our choices. By applying the thoughts, ideas, and strategies that resonate with you, you will be able to better manage your anxiety, and enjoy more fully all the good things in your life.

When I wake up with anxiety, I go through a mental checklist (more about the checklist on page 292). Within 10 to 30 minutes, the anxiety is usually gone. This is just one of the ways in which I have learned that managing anxiety is attainable.

What does managing anxiety in one's life feel like?

It feels empowering. It feels like I have a choice. It feels like I can. It feels like I have a right to be happy. It feels like I am able. And it feels like I am worthy of thriving.

Now imagine a life in which you're telling people you feel "GREAT," and you mean it!

Anxiety versus stress

People have asked me many times if anxiety and stress are the same thing. Anxiety as an emotion has a fuzzy boundary and can take on many forms and degrees. The result manifests in all kinds of effects: emotionally, mentally, in physical symptoms, and behaviours.

I would call anxiety a type of stress. Stress can come in many forms: heat, lack of water, lack of air, cold, hunger, pain, discomfort, over-stimulation, and so on.

Since publishing the first volume of *Anxiety Warrior* , I have met wonderful sponsors and people committed to serving our fellow humans and empowering and enhancing people's lives. I also heard from many people who had read the book. From their collective enthusiasm and commitment, I quickly realized that we all had much more to share, which is what led to *Anxiety Warrior: Volume Two* .

The stories in this volume are deeply heartfelt. The writers have taken the risk of showing their vulnerabilities and sharing their deepest struggles so that you, the reader, do not feel alone. Their hope is that you will feel encouraged and feel that you belong and are included.

The education information about what anxiety is and its layers is included in Volume Two. Separation Anxiety and Health Anxiety have been added.

As many of you have heard me say, "There are many roads to Rome." We just need to find the road that works for us.

**Every "body" is unique. It is important
to trust yourself. To know yourself
and know what works for you.**

Do you know what your limits are? Your food sensitivities? Environmental sensitivities? Emotional sensitivities? Physical sensitivities?

It saddens me to think that people who feel "badly" continue to feel stuck, or perhaps someone has told them they have anxiety and/or depression and they think this is their lot in life. They might try one way and if it does not work, they feel stuck with having anxiety or depression for the rest of their lives. Some feel so badly that they end their lives.

After The Anxiety Warrior Project, I learned that people were so grateful for what they called "behind the door" strategies. Many felt relieved! Clients in my private practice find hope in practical strategies. For the first time they feel that they can learn and have a chance at a wonderful life.

All the more fuel to share our resources, as most of these strategies are within reach. The contributors in this book are passionate about sharing their stories, their resources, and their successes, for which I am most grateful.

We can do this!

Notes

1   Insurance Journal 2003, as cited by the Government of Canada in *The Human Face of Mental Health and Mental Illness in Canada*, 2006, pg. 41.

2   Cited in "Teen Depression and Anxiety: Why the Kids Are Not Alright," an article by Susanna Schrobsdorff for *Time Magazine,* posted October 27, 2016; http://time.com/4547322/american-teens-anxious-depressed-overwhelmed/.

How to Use This Book

TRY, EXPERIMENT, take baby steps or put your seat belt on!

It's okay if it feels a little scary.

RISK, get muddy, have fun and try again. Be playful! *Gambaru!* (Japanese for "Don't give up!")

Remember that your life is a journey that is uniquely yours. In this book, you can decide what you want to read first. Consider this book as an offering of ideas. Put together the resources that are best for you.

The chapters have strategies and exercises that are useful suggestions for managing anxiety. The poetry is a small collection of artistic expression. The Chikara warrior stories have much strength and show how awareness, determination, practice, and giving to others matters. The Senjutsu (tactics) at the end of the book gives a list by story of the resources these Chikara warriors used ("senjutsu" is another Japanese word, meaning "tactic").

What to expect while using the book

Sometimes, learning a new skill is a struggle. The process of learning can be awkward. The awkwardness and unfamiliarity may bring on anxiety. This anxiety could be fear of the unfamiliar or familiar, the unknown, a perceived known, failure, and/or success. Consider where your awkwardness is coming from. Always honour yourself and listen to yourself. Be gentle and take your time. If you feel discouraged, try something else. With familiarity and experience comes confidence.

Build a list of the ideas that work for you. Copy the list a few times and put it in safe places. You will know where to find them.

Consider the support of a fellow reader and/or friend to check in with, and to exchange ideas and insight with.

You may find that some tools are already part of your foundation. My hope is that you continue building your resources. Others may come easily to you. The unfamiliar tools just take more practice, like any new skill. From experience I have found that as we combine the tools, their effectiveness increases exponentially.

Know that we are all unique, with unique strengths and weaknesses. Consider your strengths and weaknesses and support them with curiosity and compassion.

A useful check-in scale

I would like to introduce a useful check-in scale. I find it is helpful for both myself and my clients to have a scale for measuring anxiety: 0 to 10. By giving your anxiety a number, sometimes it is easier to identify . Zero is no disturbance, so at 0 you are calm, settled, and relaxed. As the anxiety level grows, the numbers get higher.

For example, I might feel a little jittery or nervous, maybe even excited, and that might be a 2 or 3, and is very manageable. However, I know when I reach a 4, I want to begin applying my strategies. I do not want to go higher, because then the numbers escalate quickly for me.

I know that my 10 means heart pain, laboured breathing, nausea, and so on. It is hard to come down from a 10: my thoughts do not go together, as though my circuitry was misfiring. So when I notice that I am at a 4, I begin my strategies.

Some people are fine at a 5 or 6. It is important to know your limits.

It does not does not matter if your 2 is different from my 2. What is important is that the scale works for you and you understand what the numbers and levels mean for you.

At the beginning of this book, perhaps even after reading the definitions, you may want to check in and give yourself a number from 0 to 10.

Also check when you wake in the mornings: What number would you give yourself?

Try a creative practice from *Anxiety Warrior Volume One* or pick a strategy from the contributors and then check in again. Using the scale will help you create your supports and resources. It will be a barometer for your anxiety and will give you clues as to what exercises are most useful for you.

Children who understand numbers from 0 to 10 quickly grasp this scale and can give their parents feedback on how they are feeling.

What Is Anxiety?

What Is Anxiety?

I wonder if anxiety is worse than it was 20 to 40 years ago, or if we have been conditioned to believe we must be positive, happy people and fail if we feel otherwise? Or perhaps we are anxious every day and get worn out and overwhelmed. Or perhaps we are set up to be anxious through media and social messages.

Studies suggest that our anxiety levels are generally higher than they were 30 years ago, and start earlier in our lives. The proportion of 15- to 16-year-olds reporting that they frequently feel anxious or depressed has doubled in the last 30 years, for boys from one in 30 to two in 30, and for girls from one in 10 to two in 10.[1]

Appearing below are definitions of various terms related to anxiety. Further on, I'll tell you about seven types of anxiety. Understanding the various forms and layers of anxiety is the first step in managing it.

Anxiety: Feelings of worry, nervousness, or unease, typically about an imminent event or an uncertain outcome. Feelings of concern, apprehension, unease, fearfulness, disquiet, agitation, angst, tension, twitchiness, nervousness. Mostly felt in anticipation of something happening.

Pathological anxiety, psychiatric meaning: A nervous disorder characterized by a state of excessive uneasiness and apprehension, typically with compulsive behaviour or panic attacks. When anxiety is a problem it affects our health, our well-being, and our happiness. When anxiety stops us from doing something, like going out of the house, going shopping, driving, taking a course, going to a party, or visiting family, it is a problem.

Worry: From an old English word "wrygan," meaning "to strangle." Allowing your mind to dwell on difficulties or troubles, fretting, being concerned, agonizing, over-thinking, brooding, panicking, getting worked up, getting stressed, getting in a state, stewing, or tormenting oneself. Worry tends to be repetitive.

Fear versus anxiety: Fear is something you feel when you are threatened, while anxiety is being afraid in anticipation of something happening. They both have the same physiological response in the body. Fear is when you are in the woods and a bear is coming after you. You are afraid, you must make a decision; you must run or take cover. Fear is an important emotion that has kept the human species alive. Anxiety is when you *anticipate* that a bear may come after you.

Chronic worry: Have you ever had thoughts that keep looping as they if they were on a reel, returning over and over again? Chronic worry is repetitive.

Anxiety can manifest in many ways, emotionally, behaviourally, cognitively and physically.

Physically: Sensations such as butterflies in the stomach, tightly curled toes, shaking, stiff neck, sore back, indigestion, fidgeting, picking, restlessness, increased heart rate, sweating, flushed cheeks, rash, hives, nausea, stomach ache, headaches, migraines, weight loss, weight gain, tension, stress, fatigue, exhaustion, restlessness, adrenalin, insomnia, agitation, clenched teeth, teeth grinding, locked jaw, Irritable Bowel Syndrome (IBS), chest pains, shortness of breath.

Cognitively: Lack of concentration, memory problems, negative thoughts, worst-case scenario thinking, "I can't" thoughts, self-doubting and self-blaming thoughts.

Behaviourally: Nail biting, hair pulling busy mind, looping thoughts, Obsessive Compulsive Disorder (OCD), avoidance, attention seeking, binge eating, skipping meals, lack of patience, anger, drinking, self-harming, taking drugs, stuttering, pacing, not finishing things, crying.

Emotionally: Nervousness, feelings of dread, feeling worthless, overwhelmed, feeling lonely, insecure, unhappy, confused, hopeless, defensive, suspicious, or frustrated.

Anxiety has many different layers and degrees of intensity. The more aware you are of these layers, the greater your ability to change them or manage them. Know your limits. One of my participants uses her anxiety to motivate and energize herself. For me, my anxiety is a clue that something is going on that I need to take care of. So I use a mental checklist to explore its possible cause. You can find my personal mental checklist on page 290.

I invite you to keep in mind how any of these signals may be useful and/or an opportunity. What is anxiety telling you? What is its signal to you?

Exploration and knowledge build knowledge. Soon the warrior becomes self-assured, self-confident, assertive, and positive.

Depression

The Mayo Clinic defines depression as a mood disorder that causes a persistent feeling of sadness and loss of interest. Also called major depressive disorder or clinical depression, it affects how you feel, think, and behave, and can lead to a variety of emotional and physical problems.[2]

A mood disorder is a general emotional state or mood that is distorted or inconsistent with your circumstances. Here's an example: At different times in our lives, we may suffer from grief and sadness. People with mood disorders suffer for much longer periods of time. They feel as if they cannot control their moods or emotions. If it's possible that you or someone you know is suffering from a mood disorder, consider seeking a professional assessment.

Depression and anxiety often occur together. If you are suffering from one, you are likely suffering from both. Sometimes anxiety occurs as a symptom of depression and vice versa.

We hear about depression in many different ways. It is part of being human; feeling sad or depressed happens to all of us. After a visit or an exciting weekend and the house is quiet again, you might feel depressed, though you may call it "low." Sometimes we might feel "blue" or "low" for a short time and it lifts without intervention. Feeling depressed for two weeks or more, with the loss of interest or enjoyment of any activities, may be a major depressive episode. People can recover from major depression but also experience it again. People rarely seek help for this, and even when they do it is not often identified.

Depression affects a person's productivity. People miss work and cannot work as effectively.

Here are some outward signs of depression:

+ Looking sad, dejected, or anxious, or speaking in a monotone.

+ Having decreased energy, feeling tired, having slowed thinking, and feeling restless. (Some people describe themselves as feeling numb and beyond tears.)

+ Crying and withdrawal.

+ Loss of interest in personal hygiene and appearance.

+ A lack of motivation in daily activities.

Depressed people have a negative world view; they think negatively of themselves and the future. They feel hopeless and helpless. They see events around them as evidence of personal flaws. They hold a sense of worthlessness and guilt. They say things like, "I can't do anything right," "No one loves me," "Things will always be rough," and "Life is not worth living." They feel sad, anxious, guilty, angry, impatient, and unworthy.

Thoughts are affected, due to regular self-criticism, worry, negative outlook, and difficultly in focusing and in making decisions. We might feel confused and think about death and suicide.

Physically, depressed people might feel tired or exhausted. They might eat too much or too little. They may want to sleep all the time or have insomnia. They may lose their sexual drive. Sometimes they have inexplicable aches and pains.

There are different levels of depression and not everyone will have all the symptoms at the same time. Again, if you are concerned, seek a professional opinion.

When anxiety disrupts your life, it's a problem.

Not all types of anxiety qualify as an anxiety disorder. It may feel very uncomfortable, unbearable, and, when unmanageable, very depressing.

If you feel your anxiety is causing a problem in your life, it may be beneficial to seek help. Some anxiety in life is normal. However, anxiety that disrupts your quality of life is problematic when it stops you from doing things you love, accepting that job you want, or fulfilling a dream you have.

Even though different categories of anxiety have names, anxiety can be layered. Don't worry where you may fit among the categories. If your anxiety is stopping you from doing something, seek professional help.

No matter what type of anxiety you're dealing with, anxiety can be managed by the following strategies:

✦ Explore and understand the possibility of a specific type of anxiety.

✦ Accept your anxiety as a gift, a signal, an opportunity, a message.

✦ Identify and understand the causes and triggers for your anxiety.

✦ Use the scale 0 to 10 to identify the intensity of your anxiety.

✦ Know your limits, (sleep, hunger, amount and type of stressors).

✦ Perhaps break down your anxiety into smaller layers.

✦ Manage the easy layers first, right away.

✦ Change your lifestyle to lower the anxiety.

✦ Practice your strategies.

✦ Know that you are not alone.

✦ Recognize that you can be in control of your reactions.

✦ Create your own daily routine and practice it daily, especially when you feel pleasant.

✦ If I could only give you two words from this book, they would be "awareness" and "practice." Become aware so you know what to change/modify/manage, and practice your strategies. Life is a process and a practice for all of us!

Below, we'll examine seven types of anxiety. More than one may apply at the same time, or at different times in your life depending on the situation.

1. Generalized Anxiety Disorder (GAD)

Generalized Anxiety Disorder (GAD), is the most common and widespread type of anxiety. GAD affects tens of millions of people throughout the world.

GAD is best described as an ongoing state of mental and/or physical tension and nervousness, either without a clear cause or without a break from the anxiety.

If you feel yourself constantly on edge, worried, anxious, or stressed (either physically or mentally) and it's disrupting your life, you may have Generalized Anxiety Disorder. Remember, some anxiety is a natural part of life, and it's normal to feel some degree of occasional anxiety. However, when that anxiety appears to occur for no reason or is out of proportion to the cause, you may have Generalized Anxiety Disorder.

The following are the most common symptoms associated with GAD:

✦ Constant restlessness, irritation, edginess, or a feeling of being without control.

✦ Fatigue, lethargy, or generally low energy levels (feeling exhausted or drained).

✦ Tense muscles, especially on the back, neck, and shoulders.

✦ Difficulty concentrating or focusing on tasks and/or activities.

✦ Negative thoughts — "disaster thinking."

When the mental and/or physical anxieties are persistent and don't go away, it may be GAD.

Generalized Anxiety Disorder can be very common in those struggling with other anxiety disorders, such as Panic Disorder and Obsessive Compulsive Disorder.

Separation anxiety

Separation anxiety is feeling anxious when separated from a loved one, or person, like a teacher. Symptoms might include disaster thinking about that person, avoiding activities that take you away from that person, constantly checking on that person, wanting to hang on or constantly touch that person, not wanting to go to sleep alone.

Constant restlessness, irritation, edginess, or a feeling of being without control.

✦ Fatigue, lethargy, or generally low energy levels (feeling exhausted or drained).

✦ Tense muscles, especially on the back, neck, and shoulders.

✦ Difficulty concentrating or focusing on tasks and/or activities.

✦ Negative thoughts— "disaster thinking."

Health anxiety

Health Anxiety means that someone worries constantly about their health or possible illness. This may result from having had previous illnesses, or not. Symptoms include thinking the worst of one's health, obsessed about any body sensations as possible symptoms, worries about dying and wondering if any signs of illness could be missed. Many symptoms could show up, as listed in this book. It is best to seek medical attention when physical symptoms do show up, along with therapeutic help.

2. Social Phobia

Some people suffer from "social phobia," or fear of social situations. Some degree of social phobia is normal. Small degrees of shyness in public places, or discomfort while public speaking, are natural in most people and do not imply an anxiety problem.

However, when that fear keeps you away from social settings, you may be suffering from social phobia. Social phobia occurs when the shyness is intense and the idea of socializing or speaking with the public, strangers, authority figures, or possibly even your friends causes you noticeable anxiety and fear.

If you have social phobia, public situations feel particularly painful and distressing. There can be a constant fear of being judged, observed, remarked upon, or avoided. Those with social phobia also often have an irrational fear of doing something stupid or embarrassing.

What makes this more than just shyness is that those fears cause you to avoid healthy socializing situations altogether. Those with social phobia often experience one or more of the following issues:

✦ Feeling hopeless or fearful with unfamiliar people or in unfamiliar situations.

✦ Obsession over being watched, observed, or judged, whether by strangers or friends.

✦ Feeling overwhelming anxiety in any social situation.

✦ Severe fear of public speaking, beyond what one would consider "normal."

✦ Anxiety about the idea of social situations, even when not in one.

✦ Intense issues about meeting new people or speaking up when you need to speak.

Many people with social phobia avoid any and all social situations as best they can, so as to avoid the discomfort of anxiety.

3. Panic Disorder

Panic disorder is a debilitating anxiety disorder that is different from GAD. Panic disorder is not about "panicking" in a given situation.

For example, panicking about being attacked by a bear is natural. Panic *disorder* is when you experience severe feelings of doom that cause both mental and physical symptoms so intense that some people become hospitalized, believing that something is dangerously wrong with their health.

Panic disorder is characterized by:

A) **Panic attacks.** These are intense physical and mental sensations that may be triggered by stress, anxiety, or by nothing at all. They often involve mental distress, but are best recognized by their physical symptoms, including:

✦ Rapid heartbeat (heart palpitations or irregular/fast-paced heart rhythms).

✦ Excessive sweating or hot/cold flashes.

✦ Tingling sensations, numbness, or weakness in the body.

✦ Depersonalization (feeling like you're outside yourself).

✦ Difficulty breathing or feeling as though you've taken a deep breath.

✦ Light-headedness or dizziness.

✦ Chest pain or stomach ache.

✦ Digestive problems and/or discomfort.

B) **Fear of getting panic attacks.** This may have some or all of the above physical symptoms, and may also involve seemingly unrelated symptoms, such as headaches, ear pressure, and more. All of these symptoms feel very real, which is why those who experience this fear often seek medical attention.

Panic attacks of both types are also known for their mental "symptoms," which peak about 10 minutes into an attack. These include:

✦ A feeling of doom, or the feeling as though you're about to die.

✦ A feeling of helplessness, or feeling like you're no longer yourself.

Contrary to popular belief, it's possible for the physical symptoms of panic attacks to come before *or* after anxiety, meaning that you can experience physical symptoms before experiencing, say, the fear of death. That is why many people may not associate their symptoms with anxiety, and instead associate them with the possibility of physical health problems.

Panic disorder can be very hard to control without help. Seeking assistance for your panic attacks is an important tool for stopping them, so that you can learn the techniques necessary to master panic.

You can also have panic disorder without experiencing many panic attacks. If you live in constant fear of a panic attack, you may also qualify for a panic disorder diagnosis. In such cases, your anxiety may resemble Generalized Anxiety Disorder, with the difference that the fear in this case is known.

4. Agoraphobia

Agoraphobia is more common in adults. Agoraphobia is the fear of going out in public, open spaces, or being in unfamiliar places. Many people who suffer from agoraphobia rarely leave their homes. Some can travel from home to work. Some can go to the grocery store or other familiar places but experience intense, debilitating fear anywhere else.

I had a client, a young man who was able to go to work. He was very responsible and reliable. He could go for drives in his own vehicle. He even could drive for his employer, as long as he had minimal contact with other people. His worry was that he might have a panic attack while shopping or being in any public place where people might notice that he was nervous. So he stayed home.

Many people who have agoraphobia also have panic disorder. People experience panic attacks in public places, so they start to avoid more and more places in order to avoid panic attacks.

Some people experience agoraphobia after traumatic events. They fear losing control psychologically and physically, which causes them to avoid social situations.

There are different types of agoraphobia:

✦ *Obsessive fear of socializing* with groups of people, regardless of whether or not you know them.

✦ *Severe stress or anxiety* whenever you're in an environment other than your home, or an environment where you're not in control.

✦ *Feelings of tension and stress* during regular activities, such as going to the store, talking with strangers, or even just stepping outdoors.

✦ *Preoccupation* with how to protect yourself or find safety in the event that a crisis occurs, whether there is cause for concern or not.

Your own fears are keeping you hostage, stopping you from going out and living life.

Many people experience moments where they feel vulnerable outdoors and prefer to stay safe in their homes. However, when the fear seems to continue for a long period of time, or is holding you back from living an enjoyable life, you may have agoraphobia.

5. Phobias

Phobias are intense fears of objects, scenarios, animals, etc. Phobias generally bring about disaster thinking (believing the worst will happen) or avoidance behaviours (doing whatever it takes to avoid the phobia).

An example of a common phobia is arachnophobia, or fear of spiders. Very few spiders are likely to bite and even fewer are dangerous, yet many people experience a feeling of severe dread at the sight of a spider. Other examples of phobias involve snakes, mice, airplanes, thunderstorms, clowns, blood, and so on.

Phobias are considered an anxiety disorder, even though some people can go their entire lives with a phobia and not require treatment. For example, if you have a fear of chickens but live nowhere near a farm, it is not a problem for you.

Alternatively, you may experience severe "what if" scenarios everywhere you go, including disaster thinking or feeling helpless/hopeless in public situations.

If at any point your life starts to change as a result of your phobia, then you may have a real problem. Phobias commonly cause:

✦ Excessive and/or continuous fear of a specific thing, situation or event.

✦ Instant feelings of terror when confronted with the subject of the phobia.

+ Inability to control the fear.

+ Going to great lengths to avoid the situation or object
  that causes the fear.

+ Changing and limiting life routines because of the fear.

For some people with severe phobias, the mere idea of the object
they fear (even if it is not present) causes stress or anxiety, or otherwise
affects their life.

Many people have small phobias they can manage, but if a phobia
ever starts to genuinely affect your ability to live your life, you may
need to seek professional help.

6. Post Traumatic Stress Disorder (PTSD)

PTSD is an anxiety disorder that can develop after one or many traumatic events. It can also happen over a period of time, and/or be a
collection of what we call "small t's" and/or "big T's" in Eye Movement
Desensitization and Reprocessing (EMDR; see the *Glossary*, page 298,
for the full meaning).

PTSD affects people both psychologically and physically. In most
cases, the person with PTSD is the one who experienced the traumatic
event, though it's possible to get PTSD by simply witnessing an event
or injury, or even by discovering that someone close to you dealt with
a traumatic event. Therapists can get secondary trauma from hearing
traumatic stories.

People with PTSD may avoid behaviours, events, things, and even
other people who may remind them of the trauma. Many people with
PTSD also experience issues with their emotional thinking and future.
Some feel a disinterest in or detachment from love. Others become
emotionally numb. Some feel that a dark cloud follows them. Others
become convinced they're destined to die. Any and all of these emotional struggles may be common in people with PTSD.

Symptoms of PTSD include:

+ Flashbacks, the most well-known symptom of PTSD.
  Those with PTSD often relive the trauma mentally and
  physically, as though it is happening again. Flashbacks
  come as intrusive thoughts, or nightmares, and/or night
  terrors, whether triggered or not.

✦ Triggers, which are often related to the event, such as smells, sounds, tastes, feelings, colours, and so on. A trigger can revive the memory.

✦ Anxiety and/or hypervigilance over recurrence. As with panic attacks, you may have PTSD if you experience:

✧ Regular, daily anxiety over the idea of a repeat event.

✧ Hypervigilance about certain locations and events, such as swimming pools, driving, fires, and so on.

Post-traumatic stress depletes your resources and resilience. You may be short tempered, less patient, and anger easily. Perhaps you may be startled or frighten easily, and/or have trouble sleeping.

If you suspect that you have PTSD, get outside help. PTSD can affect people for years after the event occurs, possibly even the rest of their lives.

7. Obsessive Compulsive Disorder (OCD)

Compulsions and obsessions are similar, but present themselves in different ways:

✦ *Obsessions* are thought based. They're a preoccupation with a specific thought, usually negative or fearful, that a person cannot get rid of no matter how hard they try.

✦ *Compulsions* are behaviour based. They're a "need" to perform an action or activity, often in a very specific way: as hard as the person tries, they can't stop themselves from performing the behaviour.

Those with OCD often exhibit behaviours and fears that are not only confusing to people around them, but which may also be confusing to the person with OCD.

For example, an obsession would be worrying that your friend will tire of you, while a compulsion would be feeling anxious if you do not touch a doorknob before you leave the house. In many cases, the feelings are linked: those with OCD may feel that they need to touch a doorknob, or their friends may tire of them.

You can have compulsions without obsessions, though in most cases sufferers will experience severe stress if they do not respond to the urge of the compulsion. You can also have obsessions without compulsions (such as the fear of germs), but in many cases these fears will lead to a compulsion, such as having to wash your hands over and over again.

Obsessive thought patterns

Many people with OCD go through a variety of thought processes that lead to their obsessions and compulsions. The following are a few examples of obsessive thought patterns and compulsive behaviour patterns:

✦ You find yourself "obsessed" with things that you appear to be the only one worrying about.

✦ You try to shake away those thoughts when they occur, usually by performing an action.

✦ You find that the action doesn't work, and ultimately the obsession continues.

✦ You find yourself upset over being unable to shake the thoughts.

✦ You find that the worse you feel, the more you seem to obsess over those thoughts.

Compulsive behaviour patterns

✦ You experience anxiety, often over an obsession (although not necessarily).

✦ You perform an action that appears to reduce that anxiety slightly.

✦ You turn to this action to relieve your anxiety, until it becomes a ritual.

✦ You find that you absolutely have to perform this

behaviour, or your anxiety becomes overwhelming.

✦ You repeat the action and reinforce the behaviour.

Compulsions and obsessions may appear to be very unusual, and it's possible to know that they're irrational and/or strange, but people with OCD still feel they can't control them.

There are many types of anxiety. People may experience them together, or separately in varying intensities. The next chapter discusses the many layers of anxiety.

Notes

1 These findings are from the Nuffield Foundation's Changing Adolescence Programme and are published by Policy Press in *Changing Adolescence: Social trends and mental health* (http://policypress.co.uk/changing-adolescence), which explores how social change has affected young people's behaviour, mental health, and transitions toward adulthood.

2 The Mayo Clinic is an internationally recognized nonprofit organization committed to clinical practice, education, and research, providing expert, whole-person care to everyone who needs healing. www.mayoclinic.org

Eleven Layers of Anxiety

Over the years, I have discovered that anxiety has many layers that may build up over time and which can gradually or quickly prevent us from enjoying our lives. In the previous chapter we discussed various types of anxiety. In this chapter I describe eleven of these layers—contributing factors that may intensify the type(s) of anxiety we feel.

I have also discovered, along with my clients, that examining and addressing these layers can lower the intensity of our anxiety and lower the scale. Some are easy to address. Others may require time and effort.

We can usually tolerate different stresses at the same time. However, we all have a threshold. If there are too many and we exceed our personal limit, we can quickly get into a highly anxious state. Your own experience and trial and error will show you what your limits are. As you build your skills and resilience, you will likely recover more quickly from anxiety.

The first step is to understand which layers are contributing to your particular anxiety. Elsewhere in this book we'll talk about ways of dealing with the anxiety.

1. Substances

Substances such as caffeine, sugar, alcohol, and drugs, whether pharmaceutical or recreational, can affect the brain and cause anxiety symptoms. Nicotine is known to stimulate the body and makes the heart work harder. Smokers will say that a smoke calms them. However, smokers tend to be more anxious and do not sleep as well as non-smokers. Excessive salt can stress the body. Too much salt can deplete the body of potassium, which is important in the functioning of the nervous system. It also raises blood pressure, putting a strain on the heart and arteries. Simple starches can quickly turn into sugar in the body. If you are sensitive to sugars, your body may react with restlessness, palpitations, and anxiety.

Edmund J. Bourne states in his books that there are about 5,000 chemical additives used in commercial food processing. Little is known about the long-term effects of these chemicals. Some have been known to create adverse reactions:

> *Case study:* I have a sensitivity to sugars, and at suppertime if I have pasta made with bleached white flour, I am up all night. I also have a cut-off time for chocolate and caffeine: if I have these by 2:00 p.m., my body can metabolize them. It takes my body 5 to 6 hours to metabolize the sugars. On the other hand, my brother and my mom can have coffee just before bedtime and fall asleep.

It is important to know your body and your limits.

If the brain does not have enough water, it can send signals to the body that are similar to anxiety.

Alcohol depletes the body of fluid and can induce reactions similar to anxiety. Wine and alcohol contain a lot of sugar. Decaffeinated products and green tea still have caffeine in them.

> *Case study:* A client called me, quite agitated and upset. She feared an upcoming panic attack. I asked her if anything unusual was going on in her life, and she said no. I asked how often she felt like this, and she answered, "Pretty much every day." Then I asked what she'd eaten that day. She said she felt too sick to eat. She'd had a cup of coffee first thing in the morning and then felt nauseous, so she did not eat. However, she then had about seven more cups of coffee. She also relayed that she had not been sleeping well. I suggested that she wean herself off coffee and call me in a week's time. When we connected again, she said she felt tremendously different. Her anxiety levels were lower and she was sleeping much better.

Again, know your limits.

Other food sensitivities can cause anxiety. If you suspect food sensitivities, you can get extensive blood work done to check. Ask your family doctor. You can also get food testing done through laboratories and naturopathic doctors. In my private practice, many of my clients have discovered food sensitivities. Once they have modified their diets, their moods become much improved.

Deficiencies of Vitamins B1, B2, B6, and B12 can lead to anxiety and restlessness. For healthy gut care and nutrition, read *A Naturopathic Medical Approach to Treating Anxiety* by Dr. Colette Harman, page 64. If you are concerned about supplement care and vitamin deficiencies, consult your health practitioner.

2. Physiological

Physiological conditions can mimic, trigger, or intensify anxiety. Being active is a way for many people to manage their anxiety levels. Our bodies produce endorphins (the feel-good hormones) when we are physically active, which helps to alleviate anxious feelings.

Hormone imbalance and/or thyroid imbalance can generate symptoms similar to anxiety. Being low on iron will also generate symptoms of depression and anxiety. If you are experiencing anxiety and still don't know why after reading this chapter, then ask your family doctor to run some tests to help identify possible causes. In my therapy practice, I usually ask, "What are you eating? What do you do for activities? How are you sleeping? If you are not sleeping well, is insomnia the cause or a result of anxiety, or both?" Lack of sleep can also cause anxiety-like symptoms. In this case, advice from a medical and/or mental health professional may be useful.

3. Reality

Is there something real that needs attending to, such as a pending decision, multiple decisions, finding a job, managing finances, visiting someone? Looming deadlines for projects? Upcoming performances or presentations? Exams? Moving? Interviews? Court hearings? Conversations with professionals? Doctor's appointments? Surgery? Separation? Health issues?

Here, fear, and anxiety can be useful indicators of very real issues we need to deal with. For example, are you worried about money? About paying bills? This may mean it's time to attend to your finances. Check out your bank account. Consider budgeting, perhaps debt consolidation, and/or a debt reduction program. It may mean research, and working with a financial coach. It is amazing the resources we have in our society to help with finances. I once attended a talk given by a colleague, who encouraged participants to let her provide them with a complementary session so that she could assess their finances and help them with planning. She suggested that people should do this even if they have no money to invest. She helps with planning for the future as well.

I took my friend up on her offer. I felt very vulnerable and generally embarrassed about the state of my finances. However, she had a way of making me feel comfortable, and once I got over my initial nervousness I felt better.

Case study: Sheila came into my private practice hysterical and weepy about her recent separation. She had trouble thinking and was blaming her past on her "over-the-top anxiety." She also believed others when they told her she was over the top. The truth was that she was currently living in her estranged husband's house with their two young daughters. Sheila had no private space and did not know when her ex-husband was coming or going. He did not respect her space. Her mother's support fell through when she could not secure a down payment for her on a house. Renting would trap her, adding to the time required to save for a reliable home for her and her two young children. At a "Maslow hierarchy level" (see the *Glossary*, page 300) she was being challenged. She did not know where to live and how to survive. When I acknowledged her feelings and explained what may be causing her anxiety, she drew a large breath and her anxiety lowered enough for her to think more clearly.

Case study: A few years back I bought a house and studio on six acres in the country. Moving from a bungalow in town was a shock. Many challenges lay ahead of me, and every day for two years I woke up feeling nauseous and panicky. I had trouble thinking, I was so distraught. A local real-estate firm that was managing the sale caused me undue hardships, and the original owner had not disclosed the house's many weaknesses. One winter later, I realized that my house did not feel safe; it was cold in the winter and the hydro was costing me $12,000 a year (an increase of $9,000 from my bungalow.) The roof leaked in seven places. At the studio, the pipes kept freezing. Ants were eating my home. I had little money to fix the problems. Even though I was trying to build a private practice, I realized I needed to get my finances in order and make my house safe, so that I could feel safe. I needed to make this a priority, as it was affecting my health and my personal and professional lives.

I was able to re-mortgage the house and install a new roof; I fixed the windows, resolved the hydro issue, and installed a wood stove. I finally felt safe and cozy and calm.

Perhaps you feel nervous about seeing a doctor or having tests done. It is natural to feel some nervousness. Can you accept that some situations will make you feel nervous? You may have a sleepless night or two. This is natural. Can you be kind and gentle with yourself, know that this is natural and do some self-care?

How can you nurture yourself in a difficult situation and know that it will pass? Again, be aware of your limits and notice any other sources of anxiety.

4. Overstimulation

Cell phones, texting, computers, TV, gaming, all within reason are useful. However, when we exceed our limits, the stimulation is over-whelming, causing anxiety. In this world of rapid technology, we come to expect quick responses and messages. FOMO, "fear-of-missing-out," has become a term for our fast-paced technical culture.

> *Case study:* Bonnie, a 17-year-old client, was having trouble sleeping. She reported getting 10 to 20 texts before bedtime from various friends. She was so conscientious that she felt she had to answer them all before going to bed. Of course this took long into the night. She was concerned about peer pressure and did not want to hurt anyone. Finally, she told her friends that she was shutting off her phone at 9:00 p.m. so she could do her homework and go to bed. She reported sleep-ing better and feeling better. When asked, Bonnie relayed that her friends accepted her turning her phone off.

Some people watch TV or the computer before bedtime. Many stud-ies show that the blue screen tricks the brain into thinking that it is daytime, so that it does not want to shut off. Take a break from any screen for an hour or two to let your brain settle down so you can sleep.

I could follow this advice too. Many times I am inspired to write at night, and then I cannot fall asleep for a few hours.

5. Cultural and social beliefs

A social belief is a belief that is taught as being true. This type of belief comes from sources that are part of our social structure, such as parents, siblings, teachers, neighbours, strangers, media, advertising, books, classmates, peers, teachers, ministers, and/or anyone who may have instilled a belief in you that you believe to be true. In reality it may not be true. It may or may not be useful. It may not be authentic for you.

Notice your beliefs. Sometimes they fit with who you are. However, you may be driven by a belief, thinking that you need to do something because you should, instead of doing something because it feels true and right for you. Doing something because of a belief and a feeling of "should do" can cause self-doubt, second guessing, inner dialogue, inner conflict, and perhaps anxiety. Noticing a belief helps us choose how to act. We may still follow a belief. However, at least we are aware that we are doing so.

Our brains lock onto beliefs because we have a deep-rooted need to belong. Going against a belief may mean risking exclusion. It is also noteworthy that we all have a combination of different beliefs. This can cause conflict within a family, a couple, or a community.

Cultural beliefs are passed down from generation to generation. When analyzed, they may have made sense four generations ago, but perhaps not now. Cultural beliefs come from our cultural heritage and families. Here are some examples:

✦ Canadians are known around the world as kind, gentle, and pleasant people. It is a generalization.

✦ Pre-marital sex: There are differences all over the world in how pre-marital sex is viewed. In some African tribal cultures, youths are encouraged to have multiple sexual partners before marriage to get the wandering urge out of their systems. Most North American parents do not condone sex amongst teens, although some help their teens practice safe sex, because they know that hormones are raging and teens will experiment. In many European countries sex is considered natural and part of human nature, so many families do not consider sexual relationships taboo. Many European women go topless on the beach. This is natural for them, and considered neither immodest nor a sexual provocation. A young woman visiting Canada bought a bathing suit top for the first time in her life. She found this strange.

✦ Death: Norms about death vary with each culture. The Chinese hire funeral criers to help people grieve. Mexicans celebrate the Day of the Dead, while North Americans tend to tidy up death with a closed casket, funeral and/or celebration of life, and move on. Embalming is a recent North American tradition that is not practiced throughout the world.

These are just a few examples of cultural differences.

I share this story in my workshops: A young girl asks her mother at Easter why the ham bone is removed and laid beside the ham. The mother answers, "I don't really know, my mother always did it that way. Let's ask her when she comes over for dinner." They ask the grandmother why the ham bone is cut out. She replied that that was how her mother always did it. She suggested it might be for flavour. Later that evening they visit Grannie and ask her if she knew why the ham bone was cut out. Grannie replied, "It was the only way the ham would fit in the wood stove."

Selected common beliefs

Life is dangerous.

You have to work hard for a living.

Opposites attract.

Boys are tough. Boys don't cry.

Girls are nice. It's ugly to be angry.

Canadians are gentle.

I make bad choices.

I'm ugly.

I am not relationship material.

Money is the root of all evil.

Rich people are crooks.

Blondes are dumb.

Blondes have more fun.

I'm not good enough.

Don't be too happy, in case something bad happens.

Skinny is beautiful.

Overweight people are lazy.

Good things don't come easy.

Play is frivolous.

Ask yourself if this belief is absolutely true 100 percent of the time. Then consider another perspective that may fit better for you and your situation.

6. Self-doubt

Self-doubt can be a symptom of low self-esteem. The insecurity of second guessing, or back and forth questioning of a decision, and of being unaware of your authenticity, as well as conflict with beliefs, can create worry and anxiety.

Constant second guessing and self-doubt can become a loop and create anxiety. The *Empowering Your Anxiety Warrior* section found in *Anxiety Warrior Volume One* provides ideas to help you focus on learning to release self-doubt and build your resilience, inner resources, and self-esteem.

7. Perfectionism

Wanting to be right, to do everything correctly and to be perfect are other causes of much anxiety. To do our best, expect the best, and strive for the best are all integral goals. However, to be perfect as a parent, employee, artist, or student is unreasonable and a set-up for stress and anxiety. How can you be comfortable in the striving and imperfection? Can you be comfortable in the process? In the middle of a project? In the middle of completion? In the middle of the mess? Can a project or goal be partly finished and admired? Yes, to all of these questions.

Does perfectionism stop you from finishing a book? Building a house, writing a play, taking a course, learning how to paint?

8. Negative thinking

Take a moment to reflect on the quality of your thoughts. Do you mentally swear? Whether at traffic, or others, or yourself, or the weather? Is life fair? Does it feel like things are always going wrong?

Do you focus on mistakes? Flaws? Are you critical of others? Or perhaps, do you wonder why people are incompetent? Do you complain a lot? Do others say you complain a lot?

Negative thinking along with disaster thinking can perpetuate worry and anxiety.

We discuss the impact of language in points 10 and 11 of the chapter *Empowering Your Anxiety Warrior* found in *Anxiety Warrior Volume One*. These sections show you how to be aware of language and how to change language so that it reflects your dreams and desires.

Can you consider inconveniences as opportunities? Challenges as learning curves?

9. High sensitivity

A highly sensitive person (*HSP*), also known as a person with sensory processing sensitivity (SPS), is someone who is hypersensitive to external stimuli and who has a greater depth of cognitive processing and high emotional reactivity. These terms were popularized in the mid-1990s by Elaine Aron. SPS is measured by the Highly Sensitive Person Scale (HSPS), developed by Aron.

According to Aron and colleagues (1997), people with high SPS comprise about 15 percent to 20 percent of the population. These people are thought to process sensory data more deeply due to the nature of their central nervous systems. Aron and colleagues state that high SPS is not a disorder and that it is associated with both positive and negative attributes.

Having high sensitivity as a character trait can make one more susceptible to anxiety and/or feeling overwhelmed. Those of us who are highly sensitive need to take care of our sensitivity. It is imperative that we have as resources daily practice and grounding skills.

The highly sensitive child

In my private practice I see many highly sensitive children. Is your child highly attuned to his or her senses? Does he or she have an excellent sense of smell or hearing? React more to pain?

Is your child easily overwhelmed emotionally? Or likely to withdraw when over-stimulated?

Many of my young clients want to hide in bed under the covers.

Perhaps your son has a greater depth of understanding than his peers, or even adults. Does he ask profound questions, think a lot on his own, or reflect on his experiences?

Is your daughter highly aware of her surroundings? Does she notice when small household items are moved, or minor changes in others, like a haircut?

Is your child very sensitive to other people's emotions? Does he or she notice when someone is feeling sad and try to help? Or appear to be especially sensitive to the feelings of animals?

If this sounds like your child, learn more about raising a sensitive child at: www.education.com/magazine/article/Raising_Sensitive_Child/

10. Memories

We've all experienced smells, actions, colours, touches, tastes, and sounds that trigger wonderful memories. That's because our long-term memory is linked to parts of the brain that regulate our emotional and physical reactions to situations and events. But if these sensory triggers are connected to stressful situations or events, they may cause anxiety. Sometimes just the trigger alone can cause anxiety, without us even recalling the memory.

11. Traumas

If you have experienced a recent trauma, processing it will take time. During this period it is natural to feel some anxiety. This anxiety will lessen over a few weeks until it disappears, but sometimes the brain gets backed up. Big and small traumas can get stuck when the brain has not processed, or cannot process, the trauma. This can happen over time or it can happen with one incident or multiple traumas.

A small trauma, a "small t," could result from falling over a bike, having to get stitches, or being falsely accused of stealing. A big trauma, a "big T," is catastrophic, like a car accident, a fire, combat, a death, and so on. The brain is equipped to process trauma, but sometimes it can't. Sometimes the reasons are clear, other times not. When the brain cannot process the trauma, this is called post-traumatic stress. As mentioned previously in the discussion of possible post-traumatic stress, seeking professional help may be advisable.

Check-in

Here is another good time to use the check-in scale. What is your level of anxiety, from 0 to 10? Are some of the layers previously mentioned manageable? Are you curious? Then continue reading, as the rest of the book is about resources and strategies to empower your warrior.

Empowering Your
Anxiety Warrior

Authenticity:
Is It Something We Really Want?

Elke Scholz

Being honest with oneself and a
way to self-compassion

To be authentic or not be authentic... to ourselves or each other most likely can be a cause of anxiety and/or stress. Our heads say one thing, "We should follow," however, our bodies get tense or nervous and/or debate the issue.

I question, do I speak up? I hear that we say we want honesty, however, when people are honest, the results generally aren't pleasant.

We hear about encouraging expression of self and our feelings. This sounds so wonderful and healthy, yet when we do, others in their response to our honesty and expression may hammer us down. Is it a limited perspective, lack of skill and/or fear? All of these?

I have ruminated about writing this chapter for the better part of a year. In the past I have been marginalized for expressing myself and for speaking up. Sometimes it does feel like loss, however, at this point I don't regret any of it.

Recently I attended a celebration of the full moon, and later of the super moon. Part of the discussion at these "circles" was about speaking up against oppression and marginalization. In some cases circle attendees said speaking up caused alienation and loss. So the choice in some instances was not to speak up.

What I am certain about is that I need to speak up and listen to my inner self first. To hear my self and my body and acknowledge myself. Then I can decide how I might proceed. In the first volume of *Anxiety Warrior* I provided exercises to help us listen to our bodies and to our inner knowing. If we negate our inner knowing and hearts, then this type of denial can make us sick, anxious, or stressed. Once we start to hear ourselves, we can move forward and make choices to look after both ourselves and the situation around us. These choices do not always involve speaking up.

As Canadians we have a culture and social construct of being nice, polite people. It does not matter whether one is male or female. Females generally are expected to be gentle and soft spoken. When we do get angry, we're often called hysterical, bitches, cold, or even "bat-shit crazy."

Men can get angry, however if "too much" they are considered to have "anger issues." Anyone who gets angry often is labeled as having anger issues.

Personally and professionally, I am set back when a child comes into my office who has been told that they have anger issues and they therefore think they have anger issues. In being authentic here, we are given a contrary message: "Be authentic, but only if you are nice and if you agree with me." This can be confusing. Anger is a feeling that just is. To be clear, I am not agreeing to act out in anger using poor behaviour.

Again I come back to the need to first acknowledge what is true for us. Then decide how to proceed. It may not be necessary to tell the other person about our unhappiness or dissatisfaction. Or maybe it is important to the relationship to express ourselves.

In my private practice, I've noted that even the most well-meaning, kind-hearted people don't always have the ability to express themselves in a mindful, skillful, non-blaming way.

We are generally not taught to:

+ Accept our feelings, and to accept and know our human needs.

+ Take total responsibility for our lives and choices.

+ Acknowledge another person's choices without feeling that we are giving in or giving up.

+ Accept that the other person *has the right to have their own feelings and experiences.*

+ We have a full spectrum of 100+ feelings, and 100+ universal needs.

Our unpleasant feelings are uncomfortable, hopefully inspiring us to change something. They are opportunities for introspection and lead us to growth; they are clues to what we need.

Many times, anger is the surface emotion that gets expressed. Somehow it is easier to express and makes us feel less vulnerable, at least in the moment. Anger also lets us know that something is amiss in our lives. We need anger. It is important for our survival.

In my experience, even young children know that acting out in anger towards another really does not achieve the desired result. And usually afterwards we feel badly that we acted out our anger.

I would like to ask the questions: Why do we yell? Why do we act out?

We "yell" to be heard. And we yell and resort to all kinds of aggressive behaviour, from making interruptions to physical actions that harm others, when we do not have more effective strategies for meeting our needs. Aggressive behaviour is on the scale of violent behaviour. I notice that, typically, the trend is to soften the description.

If only we could slow down to listen to ourselves, and listen to the other person. When we really listen, we might not need to yell, or to keep yelling.

Why do people accuse each other? Judge each other? And why does arguing quickly get out of hand? Why do we do things that might potentially hurt others? It's because mostly we want to be heard and we long for our needs to be met. Anger, blaming, and accusing are signs of inner pain.

When our needs are met, we thrive.
We are happy and not angry.

Communicating without anger

Marshall Rosenberg, developer of Non-violent Communication (NVC), considers anger a gift. He has won over seven international peace awards for this model. He says that when our needs are met, we thrive. When needs are not met we feel anger and many other feelings that go with that anger.

NVC focuses on three main aspects of communication:

+ Self-empathy—in this model, having a deep and compassionate awareness of one's own inner experience.

✦ Empathy—understanding what's in the heart of another person.

✦ Honest self-expression—expressing oneself authentically in a way that is likely to inspire compassion in others.

Our social constructs teach us habits of thinking and speaking that perpetuate and lead us to psychological and physical violence. NVC theory proposes that although our needs don't clash, our strategies for meeting these needs clash with each other. If we can identify our needs and the needs of others and the feelings that surround these needs, harmony is possible.

I use NVC in my personal life with my close friends and family, and it has proven to be very effective. I am not always good at it, though I can step back and think things through to proceed.

Professionally, I share this model in my private practice. Many of my clients have used it successfully for their own self-compassion, discovering their needs and how to meet those needs. Marshall Rosenberg has many accessible YouTube videos in which he teaches his model.

While NVC is mostly taught as a method of communication designed to improve compassionate connection to oneself and others, it also can be interpreted as a spiritual practice, a set of values, a parenting technique, an educational method, and a world view.

As humans we have a full range of feelings, not ever to be defended or denied. The feelings we have just are. We are all individual and will have different feelings in different situations.

As humans we all have a range of needs, these needs also vary within each of us. Again, the level of need or longing is not to be defended.

Feelings and needs are neither right or wrong. They just are and we all have a full spectrum of them.

Because we are not taught this, I notice that we tend to mix up facts with self-empathy, judgments, perceptions, and assumptions. We cycle around this and can go on for years. And rarely do we get to our and the other's feelings and needs, nor to looking after those needs.

In this model we can learn to identify the facts of a situation without blame or accusations. The model helps keep the communication clean, authentic, and true. It is a self-responsible approach.

We can feel our anger response, acknowledge it, and as Marshall says, have the "party in our imagination" of how we might feel like reacting, knowing that doing so will sabotage what we really want to happen. Once we can think reasonably again, we can work through the model to identify our judgments, perceptions, opinions, and assumptions, which are not facts.

Communication is a process. Our language is a small part. Tone, voice, body, and heart are very important.

Here is how the model works for self-compassion and then for communicating and compassion with others.

Self-compassion:

✦ When you feel a heightened unpleasant emotion (does not always feel like anger), first acknowledge your feelings and discomfort, no matter what the level is.

✦ Give yourself 30 to 40 minutes of quiet time, and use the cheat sheets / models provided at the end of this section. Even when I am feeling so unpleasant that I can only think enough to remove myself, I pull out my sheets and then reflect.

✦ Fill in the model (iii). Fill in the sections, one fact at a time. Typically we include many facts, and this clouds the process and our feelings.

✦ What is self-empathy? Example: "I wouldn't do that, I work so hard."

✦ What are your judgments, assumptions, perceptions, and opinions? (Hint: these are not facts. For instance, "They are mean, they did this on purpose, they don't care," and so on.)

✦ Then use model (i) to list all your feelings. List them all; they all matter. Afterwards, pick the strongest three or four.

✦ When a fact happens, I feel... because of my longing for... Refer to model (ii) and list all your needs; again, all needs matter. Then pick the main three needs for the fact you listed.

✦   We are ultimately responsible for meeting our own
    needs, so making a request of yourself and taking further
    reflection is how you do take care of your needs. For
    example, if you chose "peace of mind," what are ways
    you can use to create peace of mind for yourself? This
    may take some more time and reflection to answer.
    When we are able to take care of our needs, our anger
    lessens and usually disappears. When our needs are met,
    we thrive.

Communication and compassion with others

After you have completed the above, perhaps you would like to take
the opportunity to make requests of another person. Have your cheat
sheets handy.

First, ask if the other person has time to listen for 30 to 40 minutes.
Be specific about the amount of time you would like and stay close
to the time line. We get exhausted when difficult discussions go on
longer.

Through this process we can structure and introduce our
conversations.

For example, you could say: "This is new to me, I feel nervous, I
don't know the best way to say this, I want to add comments in the
spirit of growing. I really care about you and I am getting triggered."
("Triggered" means being set off or activated.)

Another example: "I have a need for/ have a longing for peace of
mind, so when the TV is on loud [a fact] I feel rattled, anxious, and
restless."

Then invite the other person to repeat, in their own words, what
they heard you say. You may be surprised that it is not close to what
you said or intended to say.

You may need to say it again, being careful not to blame. Keep it
about your feelings and needs, e.g., "This is about how I feel and I will
try again..." Stay in the model and once they have heard you, then you
might begin with what you are going to do to meet your needs.

When you make a request of the other person, be careful to consider words of requesting, not of demanding or blaming. Remember
that the other individual may refuse, or they may have some ideas
that lead to discussion.

In model (i), the request for support can be made to anyone outside
of the situation.

Model (i)   NVC WORKSHEET

Work through this sheet first so you are familiar with all your feelings and needs and already have resolved how you will meet your needs.

Ask if the other person has time to listen. You'll need about 20 to 30 minutes.

Fact/Situation: One fact at a time.		
Self-empathy	**Judgments Assumptions Perceptions and/or Opinions**	
Feelings	**Needs**	
Ask the other person to repeat back in their own words what they understood you to say. (Sometimes you may need to gently repeat your statements.)		
Request of self How are you going to meet your needs?	**Request of other** After meeting your needs, you may (or not) want to make a request. If you want, you may make a request of the other person.	**Request for support** Or you may make a request for support from someone outside the situation, e.g. family member, neighbour, friend, and/or counselor.

Model (ii)   FEELINGS LIST

(There may be more feelings not listed here, just add them, being careful that they are not perceptions. Check the perception list at the end.)

You may feel any of the following feelings:

Unpleasant Feelings List

Anger
upset
bitterness
edgy
enraged
exasperated
frustrated
impatient
irritable
irked
agitated
furious
irate
outraged
resentful

Averse
disgusted
horrified
repulsed
appalled
contemptuous

Confused
dazed
hesitant
perplexed
puzzled
torn
lost
mystified
baffled
bewildered

Discomforted
disturbed
perturbed
rattled
restlessness
startled
shocked
surprised
troubled
turbulent
uncomfortable
put down
unsettled

Disconnected
numb
apathetic
bored
distant
distracted
indifferent
uninterested
withdrawn

Embarrassed
ashamed
flustered
self-conscious
guilty

Fearful
afraid
alarmed

apprehensive
anxious
distressed
frightened
hesitant
nervousness
panicky
paralyzed
petrified
terrified
scared
tense
worried

Pain
devastated
grief-stricken
heartbroken
hurt
lonely
miserable
regretful
remorseful

Sad
hopeless
depressed
despondent
disappointed
discouraged
dismayed
gloomy
heavy hearted

troubled
unhappy
wretched

Stressed out
burnt out
depleted
exhausted
fatigued
listless
overwhelmed
restless
sleepy
tired
weary
worn out

Vulnerable
fragile
guarded
helpless
insecure
leery
reserved
sensitive
shaky

Yearning
envious
jealous
longing
pining
wishful

Pleasant Feelings List

Affection	**Glad**	pleased	content
compassionate	alive	thrilled	fulfilled
friendly	amazed		relaxed
loving	amused	**Grateful**	relieved
sympathetic	awed	appreciative	satisfied
tender	encouraged	moved	
warm	energetic	thankful	**Rested**
	enthusiastic	touched	alert
Interested	excited		alive
absorbed	grateful	**Hopeful**	energized
alert	happy	encouraged	invigorated
curious	hopeful	expectant	refreshed
enchanted	inspired	optimistic	rejuvenated
engaged	invigorated	**Peaceful**	relaxed
fascinated	joyful	calm	renewed
intrigued	motivated	comfortable	strong
spellbound	optimistic	centred	
stimulated		composed	

The following words are sometimes confused as feelings, when in fact they are perceptions, assumptions, judgements, or opinions. We still might think that we "feel" these.

Perceptions List

abandoned	criticized	misunderstood	rejected
abused	ignored	overworked	put down
attacked	intimidated	patronized	threatened
betrayed	manipulated	pressured	tricked
cheated	neglected	provoked	unappreciated

Model (iii)   UNIVERSAL HUMAN NEEDS

Adapt this needs list to best suit your wording. Use it as a guide.

Physical sustenance and security
air
food
physical safety
rest/sleep
shelter
touch
water

Emotional/ spiritual security
consistency
order/structure
peace (external)
peace (internal)
peace of mind
protection
safety (emotional)
stability
trust

Freedom
autonomy
ease
independence
power
self-responsibility
space
spontaneity

Leisure/ Relaxation
humour
joy
play
Connection

Affection
appreciation
attention
closeness
companionship
harmony
intimacy
love
nurturing
sexual expression
support
tenderness
warmth

To matter
acceptance
care
compassion
consideration
empathy
kindness
mutual recognition
respect
to be heard

to be known
to be seen
to be trusted
to be understood
understanding others

Community
belonging
communication
cooperation
equality
inclusion
mutuality
participation
partnership
self-expression
sharing

Meaning
Sense of Self
authenticity
competence
dignity
growth
healing
honesty
integrity
self-acceptance
self-care
self-connection
self-knowledge
self-realization

mattering to oneself
aliveness
clarity
discovery
learning
making sense of life
stimulation

Understanding
awareness
challenge
consciousness
contribution
creativity
effectiveness
exploration
integration
purpose

Transcendence
beauty
celebration of life
communion
faith
flow
hope
inspiration
mourning
peace (internal)
presence

Resources

❖ *Nonviolent Communication: A Language of Life* by Marshall
   B. Rosenberg, 2015. Puddledancer Press, Encinitas, CA.

Anxiety and the Body

Dr. Nick Bianchi

I have known Dr. Nick for many years. I have listened to his engaging talks and go to him for my body "tune-ups." He has an open approach and is curious about the body and what is going on in it and why. In my experience, he continues to be a life learner and is well read. Nick practices his philosophies and embodies a tender, light-hearted and humourous view of his own humanness.

— Elke

If I were to describe myself and my approach to healthcare, I would say that I am a body-worker who is fascinated with and honours the body's relationship to the mind. Chiropractors deal with the body—the bones, muscles, joints, and nerves. We realign, loosen, and adjust. We manipulate, mobilize, and massage. We restore a person's biomechanics so that they have less pain with better function. Behind it all, we look for the cause: *Why did this happen to this person? What caused their body to distort, to tighten and to seize up?*

Chiropractors have looked for the cause from the beginning and categorize it in one of three ways: a physical trauma, some form of toxic substance, or mental. Yes, mental, as in stress. Most of you will understand the connection between our mental states and our body states—a happy person smiles, an angry person clenches, and a stressed person has shoulders up around their ears.

I am not a therapist of any kind, yet if I were to become one, it would be a body-centred psychotherapist. Anxiety finds expression in the body and the body can be a cause of anxiety. Those of you who have anxiety need to know that practices such as yoga, running, and weight training are excellent methods to expose our mental patterns and change them. You should also know that our physical health can be a significant causative factor. In *Anxiety Warrior Volume One*, Elke explained the relationship between physical health and anxiety, and I encourage you to (re)read this wonderful resource. It is my hope that as I share insights into my world, it will help you to manage your situation and perhaps send you on ever-more-fruitful journeys towards greater wholeness and well-being.

> *"Why does it keep coming back?"*
> *"How did this happen?"*
> *"But I didn't do anything! I just woke up with it!"*

These are some of the common statements made by patients in my office, which I believe are similar to other chiropractors' experiences. Being a chiropractor gives me a unique perspective on the connections between healing of the body and the state of the mind. Chiropractors (and body-workers in general) have different relationships with their patients. The hands-on experience is intimate and personal, and the quantity of successive treatments allows for a sharing of a person's life challenges and struggles. This, coupled with the chiropractor's desire to identify the causes of the patient's problems, has led me to know quite a bit about anxiety both from a patient's and a clinical perspective.

Anxiety (and stress in general) underlies a significant number of problems that present in a chiropractor's office, and to ignore this would lead to incomplete treatment and, truly, incomplete healing. I have learned about anxiety from my patients, studied it academically, and have had periods of anxiety and stress in my own life as well. Anxiety affects our physical bodies, and our physical health influences our mental state, which can result in anxiety. In this chapter I will highlight these two sides of the anxiety/body connection, and provide you with some fresh perspectives on how to further manage your condition.

Effects of anxiety on the body

Anxiety is experienced in the mind but felt in the body. It triggers a stress response—a default program in our *body-mind*. I use this term as it nicely expresses the connection between these two parts of our being. We have, as a culture, separated the body and the mind for too long, and I am happy to see the re-establishment of this truth that all traditional healing arts assumed for thousands of years before we became "modern."

If you have never heard about this phenomenon, it is quite easy to feel in real time. Imagine a large, snarling bear walking into the room where you sit, right now. What would happen? Would your heart race, your eyes widen and your muscles tense up? You bet they would. Would you be fearful as to what will happen next? If you didn't become fearful at this point, you would probably have a very poor outcome.

This, in short, is what occurs in our bodies when we are anxious and/or stressed. Early in our evolutionary development, the majority of threats and stresses were physical in nature and demanded an appropriate physical response. As part of our genetic inheritance, we respond to threats and stress powerfully and immediately. In the short term, this response keeps us alive. Over time, however, it can literally kill us.

The problem today is that most of our stresses are not physical and last a long time. Furthermore, the perceived threat does not even have to be real. Having a bear in the room is an example of a real, live threat to which the body-mind would respond. However, experiencing anxiety will elicit a very similar response. In short, anxiety of the mind can lead to a racing heart, muscle tension, and chronic pain.

"How did this happen, Dr. Nick? I just woke up with it!"

Neck pain, back pain, muscle soreness—resulting from a fall, injury, sporting event or even aggressive gardening—are accepted as understandable consequences. If a person falls down the stairs and lands on one shoulder, it should hurt. However, many people have muscle tension, twists and distortions of their skeleton, pain and stiffness for reasons that, for them, are unknown. No fall, no injury, no household chores; they simply wake up to their problem. What happened? Did they just "sleep funny"? Probably not. Many times it is the proverbial straw breaking the camel's back. Stress and anxiety are common causes and/or significant factors in musculo-skeletal pain.

Anxiety will create muscle tension, which can lead to those tender knots that massage therapists love to find. Muscle tension can create skeletal imbalances leading to twists, distortions, and overall bad posture. Joints become stiff and bones are pulled out of alignment. Heart rate increases, as does blood pressure. Chronic anxiety = chronic stress, which can lead to adrenal fatigue and disruption of many other hormones, including thyroids and insulin. The ability of the body to heal is diminished and injuries can occur more frequently.

It has been claimed that stress of some sort is responsible for 75 percent of visits to the doctor. That stress may be caused by smoking, eating junk food, or anxiety. The take-home point is this: If you suffer from anxiety, then you will have physical manifestations of it, likely in your musculo-skeletal frame. It is important that you tell your chiropractor/massage therapist/physiotherapist/acupuncturist that you have anxiety, because it will help them to understand why your body is the way it is and why it is healing (or not healing) the way it is. It can also greatly alter the clinical approach when working with you.

We all want to know what is wrong with us; that is, we assume that something is wrong. Why else would we have symptoms? Sometimes, physical symptoms are simply normal and, in fact, healthy. If someone vomits food that contains toxins, isn't that a good thing? A cough that produces phlegm is a way for the body to eliminate bacteria. Symptoms may be unpleasant and we, of course, want them to go away, but they may also be a sign of health. Please don't automatically add your back pain and shoulder aches to your list of how broken you are. The physical manifestations of anxiety are a normal response. You may not be broken, and in fact may be functioning quite well.

Work with the body, not against it

> *"Great! I'm anxious and I have back pain, knots in my shoulders, and tension headaches. Now what?"*

I would suggest using a phrase other than *"I am anxious."* I think that it would be more powerful to remove the "I am" and instead say something like, *"I experience anxiety and my muscles hurt, I get headaches, and my hips are out of alignment."* It is important to distance ourselves from our anxiety, which allows us to deal with it as a separate thing rather than to see ourselves as a broken person.

It is important to distance ourselves from our anxiety, which allows us to deal with it as a separate thing rather than to see ourselves as a broken person.

A natural and common reason why patients come to see me is for resolution of their pain, tension, and aches. They want me to magically take away their symptoms and their stress, which I really can't do, but I understand their request. What I am about to discuss is very important and can be life changing. A lot can be said about it and a lot has been written, which I will reference further on. However, this will get the point across.

The question is whether a doctor or therapist should fulfill the desires of their patients to "remove" their pain. Perhaps what is needed is education and encouragement to allow the patient to go through their process and heal themselves.

I do agree that sometimes, in some people, in some situations, it is appropriate, important and essential to do what is necessary to make them comfortable and ease their suffering. However, for many people what is needed is a different perspective, one that supports growth and understanding, and leads a patient to a much more empowered place. Unfortunately, this path takes some effort and is not supported by our current culture.

What I am asking you to consider is that instead of finding a method/person to get rid of your symptoms, try instead to simply be with it and merge with them. Befriend them, and they no longer become your enemy. In martial arts one can either block an opponent's blows or absorb them and return the energy. Many performers will use their nervousness as excited energy to fuel their performance. Musicians need to become one with their instrument and athletes need to get into the flow of the game. What if instead you became curious about your symptoms? What if you sought to discover the gifts behind your wounds? What if I told you that to become an adult human being, you have already had to overcome myriad challenges, turmoils, and frustrations? Do you remember learning how to walk, hold a fork and tie your shoes? Do you recall how foreign it was for your brain to link together sounds and written letters?

I know that you already know how to be with a challenge and become stronger because of it. Now, do it with your body pain and your anxiety.

Here is a great way to bridge these two worlds. Say that you have tension headaches and you would really like someone to relax the muscles and manipulate the joints, releasing pressure, creating more ease of movement and decreasing pain. Yes, this is a good thing. However, what I am suggesting is that you adopt a different mindset as the therapy is being delivered. Instead of being passive, get involved with the healing and co-create. Be with your body, feel the tension, explore the tautness and accept the pain as a teacher. Allow the body-worker to help you to explore what your body is experiencing. Feel it, learn and grow.

What will you feel? At first you will feel more pain, then I suggest that you look for something more.

What else is there? Become curious and open. What do you experience as someone works on your body? Is the pain coupled with anger, sadness, frustration, or fear? These are common emotions, but there may be more.

Some people experience memories, recall dreams or have what they can only refer to as a spiritual experience. I recall a time when I received a leg massage—I am an avid runner and achy leg muscles are common—and came to know this experientially. As the therapist worked on my left leg I felt angry and tense. As she worked on my right leg I felt open and receptive. Both were equally painful in terms of the muscle pain, yet my internal experience was quite different.

After the massage I spent some time in contemplation and related some of what I had experienced in my relationships with others and myself. My left side pain triggered emotions that I had not dealt with in my past and present life, whereas the right side was connected to my larger self. I gained a more profound appreciation of the body-mind, and learned to make different choices from that point on. Importantly, my legs seemed to be looser than normal because I had merged with the reason why they were tight in the first place. They no longer had a reason to be tight and I was a better person having gone through it all.

The body does not lie and no, you cannot just stretch away your problems. Be mindful of the words you use with your practitioners and watch for phrases such as, *"Just fix me," "Get rid of these knots,"* or *"Just crack me here, Doc."* I understand that this may be a challenge for you, let alone your practitioner. However, like all things that require effort and focus, the fruits of your labour will be life changing, and this process will become a significant step in the management of your anxiety.

Imagine if you could adopt this perspective: *My brain is under the influence of certain chemicals that give me the experience of anxiety, my body-mind matches the anxiety by becoming tense and distorted, yet I remain well, aware, and in control of how I choose to interpret all of this...*

Body tension creates anxiety

Let's switch gears now. I have been focusing on the brain causing body tension, but how about the other way around? Can a tense body create anxiety? How can our bodies experience stress on a physical level, which leads to mental stress as well?

The brain receives input from our nervous system (the nerves and sense organs, such as taste, sight, hearing, smell and touch) to understand our environment. The brain also receives nerve input from the inside of our bodies (heart beats, muscle tension, posture, etc.). Whatever is perceived is used to create pleasure (the smell of freshly baked apple pie), disgust (dirty diapers) or stress/anxiety (mail with the words "Final Notice" on it). If the brain becomes aware of a body that is tense, stiff, and achy, it will look for a mental match to this bodily experience and stress/anxiety is a likely choice.

Because of the aforementioned stress response, our brain is hard-wired to assume that tension = threat = anxiety. How do you feel and respond after a long drive stuck in traffic? How are you when you eat poorly? Have you ever been hung over and found yourself short and snappy? What happens when you miss your workout?

One of the reasons why exercise and proper nutrition are so important is that they keep our bodies humming along in a good, healthy state. When our bodies are happy, our brains receive many positive messages and are more likely to match that happiness.

When you look for another tool to manage your anxiety, do yourself a favour and find a physical activity that you enjoy. Then get some recipes for healthy and tasty food. Your brain will thank you, your anxiety will diminish, and you will start to make even more healthier choices.

Some causes of body pain

We know that mental stress can create body pain, but how about the other way round? Common reasons why the body would experience pain, which affects the mind, include:

+ Too much sitting. Spend the majority of your day in motion and not in sitting.

+ Poor food choices. Beyond the obvious junk food, sometimes even what is considered healthy may not be good for us. Many foods are in fact inflammatory, meaning that byproducts produced when these foods break down produce inflammation inside the body. Do you think that this situation is anxiety provoking? Conduct a quick online search to learn which foods can trigger inflammation.

If you are reading this book, you are likely confronting the adversary of anxiety. Be the hero of your own life. Gather your strength, get some help, respect your adversary, meet it head on, and become a better you. The toughest battles produce the greatest stories; realize that you are in a great story!

Resources to help you take on your anxiety

Many resources flesh out the connections of the body-mind's relations to stress, anxiety, PTSD, trauma, etc. Here is a by-no-means exhaustive list, and I encourage you to peruse the Internet for other sources. Anxiety as I know it is something that we do not seek to cure or eliminate but to manage. I would to go one step further and see it as an opportunity for growth and maturation. Just like going up a ladder requires effort, the challenges in life shape us and make us who we are.

Resources

Dr. Donald Epstein, *The 12 Stages of Healing: A Network Approach to Wholeness*. Amber-Allen Publishing, New World Library, Novato, CA, October 16, 1994.

Donald M. Epstein, Simon A. Senzon, and Daniel Lemberger, "*Reorganizational Healing: A Paradigm for the Advancement of Wellness, Behavior Change, Holistic Practice, and Healing*," The Journal of Alternative and Complementary Medicine, Volume 15, Number 5, 2009.

Sherianna Boyle, *The Four Gifts of Anxiety: Embrace the Power of Your Anxiety and Transform Your Life*, Adams Media, December 5, 2014, USA.

Peter A. Levine and Ann Frederick, *Waking the Tiger: Healing Trauma*, North Atlantic Books, Berkeley, CA, first edition, July 7, 1997 (also available as an audio book).

Bessel van der Kolk, *The Body Keeps the Score: Brain, Mind, and Body in the Healing of Trauma*, Penguin Books (also available as an audio book).

Babette Rothschild, *The Body Remembers: The Psychophysiology of Trauma and Trauma Treatment*, W. W. Norton & Company, first edition, October 31, 2000, New York, NY (also available as an audio book).

Stephen W, Porges, *The Polyvagal Theory: Neurophysiological Foundations of Emotions, Attachment, Communication, Selfregulation*, W. W. Norton & Company, first edition, April 26, 2011, New York, NY.

Ken Dychtwald, *Bodymind*, Jeremy P. Tarcher/Putnam (a member of Penguin Putnam), second revised edition, April 1, 1986, New York, NY.

Anxiety Meets Compassion

Nicki Koethner

I met Nicki at a meeting of the International Expressive Arts Therapy Association (IEATA) Board, and at the Hong Kong and Winnipeg conferences. I have enjoyed her clowning performances and our fun times together. When you meet her, you will see the pure twinkling dance in her eyes that delights in the world and life.

— Elke

The jittery feeling of anxiety is uncomfortable, urging me to move outside of my body, especially my heart, and orienting me to others: "What are they thinking of me? What will they think of me? I'm a fraud. Amounting to nothing good!" My thoughts predominate, and distort what I see and hear. "I don't really listen or receive anything since I already know it all. I know how it will turn out. They will see how flawed and bad I truly am." Anxiety takes over my experience.

"I'm afraid of being judged, criticized, and attacked." The eternal pressure of right and wrong and all the "shoulds" I have accumulated throughout the years. Perfectionism driven to an extreme. "If I only get it right. If I only know what to say, do and feel. There must be a right way."

"What-ifs" and control—my constant companions. Depression and suppression not too far away either.

I want to control the uncontrollable, I don't like anyone to see me as I am. "If they only find out who I truly am, how flawed, how bad, how wrong—judgmental inside and out." "I don't like the messiness or rawness of feelings." "I don't like myself—my humanness."

"But wait a minute," Compassion says. "Anxiety, you too have gifts."

"What gifts?" Anxiety asks. "I'm not wanted or desired. I know many people know me but most want me gone from their lives. Very few accept me as a gift or see the purpose behind my existence. I'm truly hated... I knew it all along," Anxiety sighs.

"I make people sweat, and I contribute to heart disease and short-ness of breath. I bring all kind of things that are unpleasant. How dare you talk about my gifts!

"Oops, now I'm getting angry. This is very uncomfortable. I'm so sorry. I hope I didn't hurt your feelings. I told you how bad I am. Ruin-ing things and relationships everywhere." Anxiety looks nervously around.

Compassion takes a moment to answer, wondering how best to show or have Anxiety experience her loving core, her desire to feel her wholeness, and her loss of innocence that has made her so predomi-nant in human experience (especially in relationships). Compassion consults with Patience, Kindness, and Curiosity.

Compassion says, "I brought some friends with me who want to speak with you. You have known them even before you were born and sometimes you remember. They are here to assist you, and while you might not always like them, they can help you restore yourself to your original form of caring, of understanding that you want to do your best and experience the deepest form of love: accepting what is and being yourself as you are, ever unfolding and making mistakes along the way.

"Would you be open to listening to them?" Compassion asks. Anxi-ety isn't so sure; the jittery feeling is coming back, she's not quite sure what this is all about and feels the eternal dread that everyone just wants her to go away.

The heartbeat becomes stronger, thoughts are racing, hands are getting sweaty and the mind is chattering so strongly she hasn't actually heard a word of what Compassion said. Anxiety doesn't trust Compassion.

Curiosity steps in, knowing it has a lot in common with Anxiety, and says, "Come play with me. I want to know what you know. Can you tell me and show me what you like? What gets you excited?"

Anxiety doesn't know at first how to respond, then takes a breath and says, "I love to know things. I want to understand and share all that I know and really love the exchange of thoughts."

Curiosity is delighted to have found a companion who likes to know, understand, and play. Someone who could match her hunger for wis-dom and knowledge. They chatter with each other for a while, their minds expanding, creating space and recognition.

Anxiety begins to relax, feeling at home with herself, and with eagerness starts writing a book and drawing pictures.

The next morning Anxiety wakes up and is greeted by her con-stant companion, Perfectionism. Looking at her writing and draw-ings from the day before, looking at them as jumbled, scattered, not coming together, she gives up the idea that she would ever amount to anything or that anyone would find anything worthy in all the ideas that were coming through. Anxiety starts to cry, gets angry and burns almost everything that she had created the night before, and decides to put things away and go on a long walk.

Anxiety feels heavy and wants to hide once again. She would have cleaned the whole house and probably drunk a lot of alcohol or watched TV and eaten whatever she could find, especially ice cream ("I-scream"), chocolate ("Oh-so-late"; also called "procrastination") and chips ("My hips are getting bigger"), but luckily she's on a walk and none of those choices is available.

So she decides to sit at the root of a tree and wait, listening to the birds, feeling the sunshine on her skin and the air gently brushing through her hair. Anxiety closes her eyes, tired from all the thoughts and nervousness running through her veins, and gently falls asleep.

She has a dream in which she meets Patience, who is wearing a purple dress, singing and dancing, whistling, looking calm and delighted, while so passionate and free. Patience doesn't know anything about time or deadlines or what others want of her. Patience is simply herself and doesn't care that the socks she's wearing don't match and her hair isn't brushed. She had stumbled and scraped her knees and found some plants to heal the wounds. They haven't healed yet, but the singing has come back and Patience is looking for water to cleanse herself.

In this dream Anxiety meets Patience beside the lake and is startled to see her so calm and free, despite the wounds. Patience doesn't notice Anxiety at first, so absorbed is she with the reflections of the waters, resting her feet in the coolness, and gently cleaning the scars on her knees. Patience's smile disarms Anxiety right away, stripping away her usual hesitancy. "I'm surprised to see you singing and so calm when you are cleaning your wounds with the cool water," says Anxiety. "Doesn't it hurt? Don't you want to scream and run away? How come you are singing?"

Patience laughs and gently says, "I'm not laughing at your questions, I just know them all too well. I was like you, always thinking that I could be better or wanting to be someone else. I felt like I was either never enough, or too much.

"But then one day, I stopped. I listened for the first time to the rhythm of my heartbeat and breath, observed nature in all its forms, and spent time with children. I planted a seed in the ground and saw it slowly growing towards the sun. I watered it every day and saw the first green leaves growing out of the ground. I was delighted but had to wait a long time before I could experience the shade it gave when it became a full-grown tree. Whenever I look outside my window now I see a beautiful tree that attracts birds, squirrels, and insects, changes its colours with the seasons, bears fruit, and is bare in winter. I hear the wind playing with the leaves, creating a beautiful song and sometimes sending me messages, reminding me of the mystery of the universe and the inter-connectedness of everything."

Anxiety thinks to herself, "That sounds easier said than done, I surely don't have that patience. I would get bored and restless waiting that long." She feels sad, jealous, and insecure, looking away, no longer listening. She picks up a stick and pokes the ground, drawing circles and patterns, thinking of leaving, becoming hopeless: "You can do it but I never will," she says.

Patience senses Anxiety's restlessness and sadness, and realizes she has lost Anxiety's attention. Patience picks up a stick too and starts drawing side by side with Anxiety, who follows Patience's stick, seeing different patterns than her own and yet similar. Anxiety wants to stop and watch, as she thinks, "Patience knows what she is doing so I should do the same."

Anxiety is surprised when Patience pauses and looks at her with concern. Anxiety wonders what's happening, not sure what to say or do, and feels a shiver through her whole body. Anxiety begins sobbing. Patience lets Anxiety cry and then gently strokes her hair. Patience begins to sing and hold Anxiety in her arms, rocking her like a newborn baby. When the sobbing stops, Patience continues her story.

"I forgot to tell you what came before I noticed the breath and the heartbeat, and watched the seed become a tree with the help of the minerals in the soil, the water, the sun, and my loving attention. Would you like to hear?" Anxiety nods with eyes open, resting her head in Patience's lap.

"I had fallen flat on my face on cement after a night of drinking and smoking. I woke up with a stinging headache and nausea. I looked at myself in the mirror and saw bruises and cuts on my swollen face and tried to remember what had happened. I had woken up this way before, but never quite as bruised. I looked as though someone had beaten me up. I realized I needed help."

Anxiety is perplexed by Patience's story, never imagining that someone so graceful, joyful, and full of loving presence could have experienced that much pain or done what Anxiety knew too well—drinking and smoking too much, waking up with a headache and promising never to drink or smoke again, only to wake up in the same condition a few weeks later.

Patience looks at Anxiety with loving eyes and says, "That is why when I fall now, I become silent, sometimes I sing or hum, and then I just look for what I need to heal, embracing what is hurting. Sometimes I don't know what I need or how I feel, but my feelings tell me they just want to be felt. I have learned to look for water and spend time in nature and ask for help when I'm lost and confused."

Patience speaks a little more but Anxiety is falling asleep, just to wake up... hearing Patience saying, "There I met Kindness and Compassion."

Anxiety opens her eyes, finding herself leaning against the tree. It has grown darker; the sun is just going down. Anxiety isn't sure what has just happened, but while walking home hears over and over again, in Patience's soothing, loving voice, "There I met Kindness and Compassion."

Anxiety looks at her remaining drawings and writings from the night before, the ones she had not destroyed. They feel inspiring and make Anxiety smile. Some she likes, some she doesn't. Anxiety decides to be patient, understanding that things will come together when they are ready, and decides to sing, play, dance, and go to nature when she has no clue what to do next or how things will turn out.

Now when Anxiety can't help herself, seeking out habits that aren't so helpful, she speaks to herself. "I'm sorry. Please forgive me. Thank you. I love you." This is a contemporary version of the "Ho'oponopono" prayer, an ancient Hawaiian practice of reconciliation and forgiveness.

When Anxiety meets Judgment and Perfectionism, she reminds herself to laugh, not take herself so seriously, not take it personally, and use humour to write and tell her story. She also reminds herself to watch from the outside, from the eyes of her soul: "Even though I'm anxious, I love and accept myself unconditionally and completely."

Anxiety is often triggered when she makes mistakes or sees others not taking responsibility for their actions, meeting her strong allies of Guilt and Shame, Anger too, is triggered; she is filled with judgmental feelings and other ways of hiding. Guess which voice helps Anxiety along: "...there I met Kindness and Compassion."

Reflections on anxiety

Anxiety wants to know it all. She loves to plan, likes to be prepared, is suspicious, and makes sure all the bases are covered.

She struggles with trust, forgets about compassion, and gets lost in the future and in the past, losing sight of the now.

Anxiety wants to do her best—always seeking, restless. Her origin is dynamic energy, openness and curiosity, which have been shunned, criticized, misunderstood, and judged.

Anxiety loves to hang out with Fear, Perfectionism, Judgment, and Morality. She is run by many rules and regulations—the driving force of the shoulds and shouldn'ts, of right and wrong.

Anxiety was once neglected, abandoned, abused, ignored, and misunderstood, and gets reignited when these wounds are touched and triggered.

She thinks a lot and likes to figure things out.

She sometimes jumps into action and at other times is paralyzed by fear.

She predicts the worst possible outcomes and is based in past experiences. She wants to control.

Being an Anxiety Warrior

Anxiety Warrior transforms the jittery feeling into a dance, reciting and writing poetry. Walking and talking. Singing and swinging.

Anxiety Warrior has no more time for worrying, understanding that her true form is caring and loving.

Anxiety Warrior: No Worrier, No More. Imagine these lyrics sung with Bob Marley's song, "No Woman, No Cry." Sometimes just switching a few letters makes all the difference.

Anxiety Warrior opens doors of perception, sees beyond appearances and accumulates helpful knowledge for all kinds of remedies.

Anxiety Warrior is comfortable with the unpredictable, the unknowable and uncontrollable aspects of life—not taking occurrences personally and surrendering her need to control the uncontrollable.

Anxiety Warrior loves the mistakes she makes. They are signs of learning and taking risks.

Dear Anxiety Warrior readers

My sharing is a story of anxiety that is based on my own experience, as well as on what I have encountered in others and on my work as an expressive arts psychotherapist with clients, students, and co-workers. My hope is that as you read the story you might recognize your experience of anxiety and find some useful inspirations (tools) for working with this energy.

My basic tip is not to identify with anxiety. It is a sensation, a neurological reaction that is distorted energy and often rooted in conscious and unconscious beliefs/thoughts that can be channeled, transformed, and used well when you meet it with curiosity, compassion, and kindness. Humour also helps.

A simple tool for not identifying with our anxiety is to repeat this mantra: "I have anxiety but I'm not my anxiety."[1] I suggest repeating it for three to five minutes in your mind while sitting with your feet firmly on the ground. Notice if there are any shifts in your experience.

When I did this exercise for the first time, I felt lighter and more positive. Worry, doubts, and anxiety left. It might not work for everyone or every time. Try it out and see if it works for you.

Another helpful mantra is the following: "Even though I feel anxious, I love myself unconditionally and completely."[2] This is done while tapping your third eye and other places with your fingers, which can shift states of anxiety. When other emotions emerge (such as anger or sadness, for example), they might feel overwhelming. Having a guide in the process can help to hold you safe during the discomfort and possible traumatic experiences that may arise. You can find out more about tapping by looking up Emotional Freedom Technique (EFT) on the Internet.

Breathing exercises, exercising, yoga, meditation, spending time in nature, walking, running, swimming, etc. can all help to change the physiology of anxiety. Find out what best works for you.

Remember that life wants you to show up, be present and laugh about yourself. If you can't, be forgiving, gentle, and compassionate with yourself.

If you are dealing with lots of anxiety that keeps you up at night, makes it hard to concentrate or complete tasks, causes panic attacks, PTSD, Obsessive Compulsive Disorder, or other forms of anxiety disorders, consider seeking professional help. The non-judgmental presence and gentle guidance of another can support the nervous system tremendously.

Notes

1   Adopted from Roberto Assagioli's psychosynthesis work: *"I have a body but I'm not my body. I have a mind but I'm not my mind. I have feelings but I'm not my feelings."*
2   *WHEE for Wholistic Healing Workbook*, Daniel J. Benor, MD, ABHM (Association of Behavioural Healthcare Management). (Wholistic hybrid adopted from EMDR and EFT), Wholistic Healing Publications, Medford, NJ. Revised 2006.

A Naturopathic Medical Approach to Treating Anxiety

Dr. Colette Harman

I lived in Kincardine 30 years ago and that is where I first met Colette. When she graduated as a Naturopathic Doctor I took my son to Toronto to see her. Within three days his severe asthmatic symptoms disappeared and he could enjoy a normal life as a child. Recently, she wrote a few books on Managing Anxiety and she also teaches a six-week program. I am delighted that our paths are travelling together again.

— Elke

In my over 25 years as a naturopathic doctor, I have successfully treated numerous people, as well as myself, for anxiety and depression. As a naturopathic doctor it is not enough just to find a "natural remedy" to replace a "pharmaceutical drug" for my patients, but to treat the underlying causes of my patients' illnesses. Almost without exception, one of the underlying causes of anxiety and depression in these patients involves dysfunction, disease, imbalances, or other problems related to digestion and gastrointestinal health. Why is that?

Gut health and anxiety

Much recent research indicates that the health of the digestive system and the microbiome is closely linked to our emotional health and well-being. What is the microbiome? The human body contains trillions of micro-organisms (e.g., bacteria, fungi, yeast, viruses, parasites, etc.) known as the microbiota, and the microbiome refers to all the genes contained within these microbes. However, the terms microbiota and microbiome tend to be used interchangeably. Bacteria make up the majority of these microbiota by weight, and viruses by number. You may think that it is bad for a human body to have all these viruses and bacteria living in it all the time, but the truth is that the body requires these organisms for optimal functioning.

Health problems arise when the balance of these microbes is thrown off as a result of gastrointestinal infections, antibiotics, oral contraceptive pills, steroid medications, proton pump inhibitor medications prescribed for indigestion and acid reflux, nutrient deficiencies, food allergies and intolerances, poor diet, and stress. Each individual's microbiome is unique, like a fingerprint, and is essential for the proper functioning of the body due to its impact on digestion, aging, moods, immunity, and cognitive function.

Many scientists now think of the microbiome as an organ in and of itself. When this organ is unhealthy, it can cause anxiety and depression. Research shows a complex interaction between the microbiome and the brain. The gut microbiota can regulate brain chemistry, the experience of anxiety and stress, and even memory.

Dr. Natasha Campbell-McBride, in her book Gut and Psychology Syndrome (GAPS), goes into great detail on the research between intestinal health and neurological and psychological conditions, including anxiety and depression. The health of the digestive system, which is composed of the mouth, esophagus, stomach, small intestine, colon and anus, is directly linked to brain health. During early fetal development, both the gut and the primitive brain develop from the same clump of embryonic tissue. When this tissue divides, one piece grows into the central nervous system or CNS (brain and spinal cord); the other section becomes the enteric nervous system (ENS).

The enteric nervous system is embedded in the lining of the gastrointestinal tract. There are 500 million nerve cells in the digestive system. This is five times more than the spinal cord. Due to its incredible complexity, the ENS has been described as the second brain. The vagus nerve is the longest of all the cranial nerves and creates a direct connection between the brain and the gut. Within the gut lie 90 percent of the body's serotonin and 50 percent of the body's dopamine. The serotonin and dopamine housed in the gut act as a neurotransmitter, sending messages between nerve cells and helping to regulate mood, sleep, and learning and can influence our state of well-being.

The vast number of anxiety and depression sufferers have some form of digestive dysfunction. Examples of poor digestive function include constant bloating and flatulence, indigestion, heartburn, acid reflux, queasiness and nausea, and bowels moving less than once per day or more than three times per day. Bowel movements should be well formed with no evidence of food particles. Should any of the above symptoms of digestive dysfunction occur frequently—an average of one to two times per week—then these digestive imbalances may be affecting your emotional health.

As mentioned before, gastrointestinal infections, poor diet, medications, nutrient deficiencies, food intolerances and allergies, plus stress, can cause an imbalance in the microbiota, leading to a reduction in the proper functioning of the digestive tract and causing low grade inflammation. This can hamper production of serotonin and dopamine, which in turn can adversely affect emotional health.

One of the best ways to support the digestive health and promote gut healing is by modifying the diet.

Foods to decrease or avoid

The most common offenders are gluten grains (wheat, rye, oats, barley, spelt), casein and lactose (the protein and carbohydrate components of dairy, respectively), and soy and sugar.

In some individuals, corn, and other gluten-free grains (rice, millet, quinoa), plus nuts and seeds, may also be problem foods.

All refined foods should be eliminated, as well as excess alcohol and caffeine.

Hydrogenated fats such as margarine and shortening are toxic to the gut as well as all heat processed vegetable oils, including corn oil, safflower oil, and sunflower oil.

Processed meats such as wieners, sandwich meats, sausages, etc., with their high nitrate content, can be problematic for many.

Following an elimination diet is a time-honoured way of determining your intolerances or sensitivities to these foods, though it does take time. Tests such as the ELISA (Enzyme-linked Immunosobent Assay) blood test can provide more insights into which foods to avoid. (ELISA is an immunological assay technique that makes use of an enzyme bonded to a particular antibody or antigen.)

At this point it must seem that there are hardly any foods left to eat, right? Well, look below for a list of all the foods, provided you are not allergic, intolerant or sensitive to them, that you can eat and which will help your mood.

Foods to increase

Greatly increase your intake of vegetables: aim to have seven different types per day, in a rainbow of colours such as green, yellow, orange, red, and white. The fiber in vegetables helps to support the growth of beneficial bacteria, or "probiotics."

Adding fermented vegetables such as sauerkraut and kimchi (made from cabbages) can also help add beneficial bacteria to the digestive tract.

Always drink lots of water—1.5 to 2.0 litres per day—as it helps flush toxins (the by-products of inflammation) from the body.

Healthy fats from pasture-fed animals, including butter and lard, oils such as organic coconut oil, organic expeller-pressed hempseed oil and flaxseed oil, extra-virgin olive oil and omega 3 oils from fatty fish are essential for optimal emotional health. Basically, fats make us feel happy. Decades of promoting low-fat diets has resulted in a lot of depressed and overweight people. Fat is your friend.

If you find that your current diet consists of a vast majority of the "avoid" foods and you feel overwhelmed, I recommend you start adding more veggies and water to your diet and then gradually decrease the worst culprits for mental health, such as dairy, wheat, sugar, and alcohol. The more gradually you decrease the problem foods, the more permanent these dietary changes will become. Remember, you don't have to make all the dietary changes at once as you may find you feel much better just by implementing some of the guidelines.

Just take it step by step and you'll reach your goal.

If you feel motivated to make significant dietary changes, there are several dietary programs that complement this approach to eating. These include the ketogenic, Atkins, Paleolithic (paleo), and Gut and Psychology Syndrome (GAPS) diets. Below you'll find a brief summary of each.

The ketogenic diet

Variations of the ketogenic diet have been around for ages. Basically, the diet involves high fat, moderate protein, and low carbs. Recent research indicates that this approach to eating results in dramatic weight loss and increased energy and mental acuity, and has been shown to have a dramatic effect on improving moods. In fact, it appears to greatly improve brain health: for example, people with epilepsy may experience far fewer seizures. This diet may also significantly reduce symptoms associated with Alzheimer's and Parkinson's diseases. The key is to limit carbohydrate intake to around 20 grams, certainly no more than 50 grams per day, increase fat intake to 150 to 200 grams per day, and maintain a moderate protein intake of about 75 grams per day. Following these dietary guidelines induces a state of ketosis, whereby the liver replaces carbs by breaking down fats for energy and producing ketones, which are used as fuel by the cells of the body. These can be measured in the urine with specific dipsticks. As long as water intake and salt intake are maintained at a high level, the state of ketosis is generally well tolerated.

The Atkins diet

This diet was developed in the 1960s and 1970s by internist and cardiologist Robert Atkins to help his heart patients lose weight quickly before surgery and to maintain the weight loss after. Initially, the Atkins diet reduced all carbs including vegetables, with the goal of the individual going into ketosis. Recently, the Atkins diet has been modified so that the net carb intake ranges from 20 to 40 grams per day. There is no limit on the intake of fat and protein, but a high intake of both is encouraged.

The Paleo diet

Also known as the caveman diet, the Paleo diet is based on the understanding that Palaeolithic humans consumed food available to them as hunter-gatherers. This means they ate what they could hunt and fish, including animal protein, seafood, and eggs, as well as foods that they could gather, including herbs, vegetables, fruits, seeds, and nuts and their oils. Foods to avoid are those not eaten by cavemen, including grains, legumes, sugars, and dairy. Anxiety disorders are improved in many who follow this diet.

The GAPS diet

The GAPS diet, an acronym for Gut and Psychology Syndrome diet, is most commonly used to treat inflammatory bowel disease, leaky gut syndrome, autism, Attention Deficit Hyperactivity Disorder (ADHD), depression, anxiety, and autoimmune disease. Much research indicates that grains can aggravate inflammatory bowel disease. This diet is based on the Specific Carbohydrate Diet devised by Dr. Sidney Valentine Haas in the 1920s to heal digestive diseases and dysfunctions.

By healing the gut you also heal the brain and can resolve anxiety and depression. Foods to avoid include all processed foods, all grains, processed sugar, starchy vegetables, artificial chemicals and preservatives, and conventional meat and dairy products. Permitted foods include steamed non-starchy vegetables, wild fish, organic meats, eggs, fruits, healthy fats, and probiotic rich foods. This diet may improve digestive disorders, anxiety, and depression.

There are many other digestive and nervous system disorders that can underlie anxiety and depression. I highly recommend consulting a naturopathic doctor or a functional/orthomolecular medical doctor (who specializes in nutritional supplementation) to diagnose and assist with the following conditions:

✦ Digestive problems due to the deficiency of betaine hydrochloride production in the stomach and/or the deficiency of digestive enzymes from the pancreas. Often, supplementing with HCl (hydrochloric acid) is essential to augment the production of stomach acid needed to activate the enzymes that digest protein. Additionally, supplementing with broad spectrum digestive enzymes that contain lipase to digest fats, protease to digest proteins, and amylase to digest carbohydrates can really enhance and improve functioning of the gastro-intestinal tract. Digestive enzymes break down foods that you eat into single molecules that your body can use. After age 40, our ability to adequately produce these digestive juices and enzymes decreases, and often supplementation and following the aforementioned dietary suggestions are necessary to enhance proper digestion of foods and reduce inflammation in the digestive tract. This often results in improved mood.

✦ An imbalance of the microbes in the microbiome corrected by replenishing the "good" bacteria with probiotics and by killing off the "bad" bacteria, parasites and yeast overgrowth in the gut. Specialty stool, urine, and blood tests can help determine which organism imbalances are present. By correcting these digestive dysfunctions, many, if not most, cases of anxiety will resolve completely.

Supplements and natural remedies for anxiety

Finally, your naturopathic doctor or functional/orthomolecular medical doctor may prescribe any of the following supplements, herbs, or homeopathic remedies to help successfully resolve your anxiety. Below is an excerpt from my eBook, *The Guide to Natural Treatments for Anxiety and Depression*. Again, it is always recommended that you be evaluated by a qualified healthcare provider before using any of these supplements and remedies. The following information is for educational purposes only and it meant to inform you of the various options available.

Nutritional supplements

There are many nutritional supplements that can help treat and reduce anxiety, such as amino acids, vitamins, minerals, and fatty acids.

✦ *Amino acids* are the essential building blocks of protein. Protein plays a crucial role in almost all the biological processes in our bodies. The human body requires 20 amino acids for optimal functioning, of which 9 are essential and must be obtained through one's diet.

✧ *Tryptophan* is the precursor to the neurotransmitter serotonin, which has been shown to elicit feelings of calmness and relaxation. This amino acid can also help improve metabolism and sleep patterns. The most common means of taking a tryptophan supplement is in the form of 5-HTP (5-Hydroxytryptophan). It is generally considered safe to take while pregnant or breastfeeding.

✧ *Glutamine* is derived from glutamic acid. Glutamine is required to synthesize GABA (gamma aminobutyric acid), a neurotransmitter that helps relieve anxiety and stress and induce feelings of calm and tranquility. GABA enhances serotonin in your brain (mostly a good thing); it also tends to reduce other neurotransmitters (adrenaline, nor-adrenaline, dopamine). Some may find it a bit too sedating. Though it is generally considered safe, a pregnant or breastfeeding woman should check with a qualified healthcare practitioner before taking it.

✦ Vitamins and minerals

　✧ *B Complex*, especially Vitamin B6 (pyridoxine), appears to have a calming effect on the nervous system as it converts tryptophan, the amino acid, into serotonin, a neurotransmitter that helps promote a stable and balanced mood. Vitamin B1 (thiamine) can boost mood and memory. Vitamin B3 (niacin) can also produce serotonin. Vitamin B5 (pantothenic acid) creates a natural chemical that can lead to the production of many neurotransmitters. B9 (folic acid) helps balance neurotransmitters. A deficiency in Vitamin B12 may lead to feelings of anxiety and stress. A good B-complex should include all the essential B vitamins.

　✧ *Vitamin C* is required for proper functioning of the adrenal glands and brain chemistry. In larger doses, Vitamin C has a tranquilizing effect that may decrease some anxiety. If Vitamin C users take a compound containing bioflavonoids, there can be reduction in stress as well. Vitamin C is a beneficial antioxidant that keeps the central nervous system functioning smoothly.

　✧ *Vitamin D3* has been shown to greatly reduce depression, especially as it relates to Seasonal Affective Disorder (SAD) also known as the "winter blues." Lack of sunshine in the winter months can definitely cause depression and anxiety, therefore taking supplements, particularly in the winter months, is recommended.

✧ *Magnesium* is a mineral with an affinity for the nervous system. This essential mineral helps to calm and relax the nervous system while keeping one energized. It is also a powerful muscle relaxant and can relieve muscle cramping. Additionally, it can help resolve digestive difficulties such as constipation.

✧ *Calcium* is a mineral and a natural tranquilizer. When taken with magnesium and Vitamin D, it can relax and calm the nervous system.

✦ Essential Fatty Acids, or EFAs, are required for good health and must be ingested because we cannot synthesize them. Only two fatty acids are known to be essential for humans: alpha-linolenic acid (an omega-3 fatty acid) and linoleic acid (an omega-6 fatty acid).

✧ *Evening primrose oil* is an omega-6 fatty acid that contains an essential fatty acid known as gamma-linolenic acid (GLA). Once taken, GLA can have a calming effect and be helpful with anxiety and depression associated with PMS (Premenstrual Syndrome).

✧ *Fish oils and flaxseed oil* are both examples of omega-3 fatty acids, and deficiencies have been noted in people who have both anxiety and depression. Omega-3s have an anti-inflammatory effect on the brain, which is believed to help resolve anxiety and depression.

Herbal remedies

There is a wealth of herbs that can help treat anxiety. Generally, these herbs are safe to use. However, it's always recommended that you consult a qualified healthcare practitioner before beginning any herbal treatment.

✦ *Kava-kava* (Piper methysticum) comes from the western Pacific islands. The roots of the plant are used to produce a drink with both sedative and euphoriant properties. Kava is said to elevate mood, well-being and contentment, and produce a feeling of relaxation. Several studies have found that kava may be useful in the treatment of anxiety, insomnia, and related nervous disorders.

✦ *Passionflower* (Passiflora incanata) acts as a non-drowsy, natural sedative that relieves intermittent nervousness, anxiety, and panic attacks. Rather than knock you out or make you sleepy, passionflower will make you feel emotionally balanced. It won't give you a hyper, excited or happy feeling. Instead, passionflower will help to prevent wide swings in mood and reduce exaggerated emotions. Passionflower is also an effective treatment for insomnia.

✦ *Chamomile* (Matricaria recutita) is used to calm nervousness, both in the mind and the stomach. It can reduce digestive discomforts and improve appetite in people dealing with a lot of stress. Chamomile is also popular for treating anxiety in children.

✦ *Hops* (Humulus lupulus) are useful for more than just beer. Hops have a long history of medicinal applications. They are used to fight the discomfort of anxiety, restlessness, and insomnia. Part of the reason why we enjoy beer could be the calming effects of the hops.

Homeopathy

As a system of medicine, homeopathy has been practiced success-fully around the world for over 200 years. It is a natural system of medicine that uses highly diluted doses of substances to stimulate the body's own healing mechanism to promote health. As such, homeo-pathic remedies are quite safe to take. However, consulting a quali-fied healthcare practitioner is always recommended before using any homeopathic treatment.

✦ *Aconitum* is an outstanding remedy for treating acute panic attacks that are accompanied by intense fear and anxiety with marked restlessness, much shortness of breath, heart palpitations, and flushing of the face.

✦ *Gelsimium* is another great remedy for anxiety where the person has feelings of weakness, trembling, and mental dullness, and can include being "paralyzed by fear." This is an excellent remedy for stage fright, anxiety before a test or a visit to the dentist, or any stressful event. Chills, perspiration, diarrhea, and headaches will often accompany the nervousness.

✦ *Kali phosphoricum* can help a person who has been exhausted by overwork or illness and feels a deep anxiety and inability to cope. The person is jumpy and oversensitive and may be startled by ordinary sounds. Insomnia and an inability to concentrate may develop, increasing the sense of nervous dread. Eating, warmth, and rest often bring relief.

✦ *Lycopodium* can help individuals who feel anxiety from mental stress and suffer from a lack of confidence. They can be self-conscious and feel intimidated by people they perceive as powerful, and yet may also swagger or be domineering toward those who they feel are inferior to themselves. Taking on responsibility can cause a deep anxiety and fear of failure, although the person needing lycopodium usually does well once started on the task. Those who require lycopodium often experience a craving for sweets and suffer flatulence and bloating as a result.

These are just highlights of the many different nutritional supplements, herbal medicines, and homeopathic remedies available to treat anxiety. Having said that, it is always recommended that you consult a qualified healthcare practitioner before starting any of these treatment approaches. Though they are generally safe and well tolerated, it is best to be under the care of a practitioner who can prescribe appropriately when indicated. Depending on each individual's situation, the outcome from the healing process can be sudden and profound, or slow and steady.

For more information, please go to my web site www.Harmany-WellnessSolutions.com where you can read my blogs and purchase my eBooks, *Anxiety and Depression: Six Simple Steps to Effectively Cope* and *Guide to Natural Treatments for Anxiety and Depression*.

Tea and Stress

Craig Denstadt

Craig is one of the wonderful people that I am blessed to have met because of The Anxiety Warrior Project. Someone in the community said to me, "You need to meet him and tell him about The Anxiety Warrior Project. *He very much supports empowering people. When you meet him, his love for tea is evident here." We are so delighted that he brings his teas to the community for us to enjoy.*

— Elke

Have you ever had that moment when your boss is yelling at you, and you just want to go crawl into a corner and hide? How about getting into a fight with your brother and reaching a point where you just can't stop shaking? How about just driving home and thinking about having a panic attack and then it happens? Well I have, and I didn't have any way of dealing with it. I thought I was going to die. My story started when I was 27.

When I was a young man, I had it all. I was popular in school, I was a top ranked swimmer in Canada, I had the cutest girls after me. I never thought it would end, and boy was I wrong. My swimming career was done by the age of 19 because I thought partying was more important and I didn't think I could do anything more with that part of my life. I gave up a chance to go on in school because I was selfish and all I wanted to do was have a good time. I figured I had it good because my parents had a family business and all I had to do was show up and work and someday I would take it over and be a rich man. Simple, right?

There were little signs along the way, but just like everyone else I didn't pay attention to them. Well, something finally got my attention one summer afternoon in 1998.

I was on my way back to my cabin in the woods where all of my fun times had happened, when all of a sudden I felt this pain in my chest—like I had an elephant sitting on me. I had never felt pain like this before. From my training as a lifeguard when I was young, I thought I might be having a heart attack. I quickly turned my car around and drove the one minute back to my parents' house. It sure felt like the longest minute of my life.

As I wheeled into the driveway, I thought to myself that if I got out of the car, I would not make it into the house. So, I decided to honk on the horn. That felt like the second longest minute of my life. Finally my parents came out and I told them about the pain I was feeling. I wanted to go to the hospital right away. My mom, who was a nurse, agreed and we drove off to Bracebridge.

On the way I was thinking that this could be it, so I told my parents I loved them. All of a sudden I burped and the pain went away. After undergoing tests that night and over the next few weeks, I discovered that I was not dying. I was diagnosed with a hiatal hernia and acid reflux (gastroesophageal disease). With a few changes in my diet and my life choices (smoking, pop, alcohol), I thought I had it all figured out. But I continued having problems.

I started having panic attacks, but I didn't know what they were, or why. I thought at the time that they were side effects of my hernia and would go away. Instead, they just got stranger.

I changed everything in my life. I improved my diet, quit alcohol, started swimming, and more. Eventually my attacks went away because of all the good things I was doing for my body. But like most people I went back to my old crutches. I guess I thought I was still unbreakable and therefore I could do what I wanted.

After battling all of my demons a second time, I realized I was fighting the wrong demon all along. The demon I needed to beat was inside my head. I started to think differently about what might be causing my attacks, and what I needed to do, on top of my health choices. Was it a fix? Yes and no, but it made it easier to deal with the problems I was having. Since those days I have only had a couple of panic attacks, so I see it as a success. I realize now that it is a battle that I have to deal with every day, and one of the ways I deal with that is with tea.

Warning: all of the opinions you will now read are for information only. Please contact your medical professional before starting any of the herbs listed below. I am not a doctor, just your local tea store owner.

Green tea

Tea is such a versatile beverage in that it has many great healing properties. It is high in antioxidants that fight free radicals in the body, it is rich in chlorophyll to help detox your organs, it helps fight off cancer, it repairs the body at the cellular level, and yes, it even helps reduce stress.

You're probably wondering how something with caffeine could help with stress. Well, tea has something in it called theanine. This amino acid promotes alpha waves in the brain, which are linked to relaxation. But don't drink too much, or at least drink decaf tea.

Black tea

A daily cup of black tea can help you recover from stress, as it has an effect on stress hormones in the body. Drinking four to six cups a day will help lower levels of the stress hormone cortisol in your blood. Black tea does not lower stress, but it does help to bring hormone levels back to normal after a stressful event.

Chamomile

Another great tea to help with stress is chamomile. Many people turn to chamomile to help them relax, since it helps soothe the stomach and decreases mild anxiety. It is also safe for children, although prolonged use is not recommended for anyone. Chamomile can also help stimulate appetite lost due to stress. In addition to drinking the tea, people can add chamomile to a warm bath for increased relaxation.

Valerian root

Valerian root is unique in that, while it is not intended for anxiety, many people find that the calming nature of valerian is extremely effective for soothing anxiety symptoms. Valerian's traditional use is as a sleep aid. Many people use valerian root to help them get to sleep when they're suffering from insomnia. But those same calming properties may have an effect on anxiety as well. In this case, valerian is dealing with anxiety symptoms directly, not the anxiety itself. You will still have anxious thoughts, but those thoughts won't create as many physical symptoms. Physical symptoms often lead to more mental symptoms, so you may still find that your mind wanders less, as a result of both the lack of tension and the tiring of your mind and body.

Valerian root should be taken carefully until you know how it affects you. The tea should be taken at night at first to see if it helps aid your sleep. If it is providing you with the effects you'd hoped for, try taking it during the day, but make sure to avoid driving until you know how fatigued it makes you feel. It should not be used by children under 12.

Lemon balm

Lemon balm is another great option to help with stress. It helps soothe your nervous system to make you feel less nervous, anxious, or upset. Lemon balm also may help reduce headaches. It is best served steeped as a hot tea for 15 minutes, or as an iced tea.

Kava

Kava is arguably the best herb for treating moderate to severe anxiety. Many studies have shown its effectiveness for anxiety and stress. Some herbal remedies ease the symptoms of anxiety, but kava might actually reduce anxious thoughts. There are some concerns about the safety of kava, so even though a cup of kava tea probably won't hurt you, it is still advisable to talk to a doctor.

Passionflower

On my long list of herbs to try is passionflower herb. It is a mild natural sedative and may help with severe anxiety, but is recommended for mild to moderate anxiety. The herb is known to decrease muscle tension and calm the nerves. It can also help with headaches and sleep problems.

Blue vervain

Another herb that will help with sleeping troubles and calming the nervous system is blue vervain. Research has shown that it can be effective against certain nervous conditions, but it should not be used for long periods of time.

Catnip

If you have cats, try stealing their catnip! Cats rarely seem stressed, or nervous, perhaps because the herb fights symptoms of anxiety. It can also reduce muscle tension, while providing mild stimulation. If your troubles are making it difficult to fall asleep, try catnip in a tea before bedtime. It could also help if lack of sleep is giving you headaches. Even people with severe anxiety may benefit.

Hops

A main ingredient in beer, hops are also used in teas to help calm the nerves and smooth out stress. They can also help with insomnia, indigestion, and headaches. If your stress level has weakened your immune system and you end up with a fever, hops could help with that, too.

Lavender

The intoxicating and safe aroma of lavender may be an "emotional" anti-inflammatory. In one study, Greek dental patients were less anxious if the waiting room was scented with lavender oil. In a Florida study, students who inhaled lavender oil scent before an exam has less anxiety, although some students said it made their minds "fuzzy" during the test.

In one German study, a specially formulated lavender pill (not available in Canada) was shown to reduce anxiety symptoms in people with Generalized Anxiety Disorder (GAD) as effectively as lorazepam, an anti-anxiety medication in the same class as diazepam (Valium).

Hawthorne

Originating in Europe and England, hawthorne has both a calming and nourishing effect on the cardiovascular system. It can have a special gentle relaxing effect on the vascular system in people who have higher blood pressures due to stress hormones.

Hawthorne contains healthy plant chemicals called flavonoids that help keep the blood vessels strong. It may also balance total cholesterol, triglycerides, and bad (LDL) cholesterol as well. Some studies also showed it may even help in congestive heart failure.

It is safe enough to take for long periods of time. The most appropriate person would be someone who has demonstrated heart and cardiovascular problems and is under a lot of stress. You can use it as a tea by itself or with other calming herbs like chamomile.

Siberian ginseng

Eleutherococcus comes from Siberia, as well as from the northern regions of Korea, Japan, and China. Commonly called eleuthero, this herb is not considered a true ginseng because it does not belong to the same genus plant family.

Eleuthero tea contains triterpenoid saponins, which are substances that have a beneficial effect on the body when it is stressed. Siberian ginseng tea improves blood circulation and enhances mental and physical prowess. It also regulates the amount of stress experienced. This herb may also help the immune system fight common viruses like the rhinovirus, respiratory syncytial virus, and influenza.

This hardy plant is known to survive brutal Siberian weather conditions. Many plant experts believe it can confer this strength to those of us who take it. Human studies seem to support this idea.

Take this herbal tea in the morning and/or afternoon. For best effect, it helps to take it for six to eight weeks, and then pause for two weeks before restarting.

The person who benefits the most from Siberian ginseng is a stressed person with a low-functioning immune system, who may have an unhealthy cardiovascular response from stress (e.g., a Type A personality), including higher blood pressure and heart rates.

Ashwagandha

An herbal medicine grown in Africa, the Mediterranean, and India, ashwagandha is an adaptogen. This class of herb helps the body fight stress by reducing the production of stress hormones that stimulate the fight-or-flight response. This adaptogenic quality can help the body relax and stay strong. It also is a potent antioxidant.

Ashwagandha contains a chemical called ashwagandholine alkaloid, which has a mild relaxant, tranquilizer-like effect on the central nervous system.

It is delicious before bed. Mix about 1 cup of boiling milk (cow, almond, rice, soy, or oat milk) with a half-teaspoon of the powdered herb or the dried leaves. Let the mixture steep for about 15 minutes and cool. Strain and then drink. Ashwangandha is known to be quite safe in the short term of a few weeks.

Ashwangandha is best for people who are nervous and exhausted after having undergone a lot of physical and emotional stressors. It's also excellent at bedtime for people who have insomnia. It can be used as an immune stimulant in patients with low white blood cell counts, so people who recently have undergone the stress of radiation or chemotherapy would do well drinking the tea during the day to rejuvenate their body.

Basil tea (tulsi herb)

The health benefits of tulsi are due to the active ingredient, Eugenol, in the leaves. Tulsi also contains ursolic acid and carvacrol, both of which have anti-microbial properties. Tulsi tea is rich in antioxidants, which help the body fight free radicals that are responsible for causing various chronic degenerative diseases. According to studies, tulsi helps in maintaining the normal levels of cortisol in the body, which is also known as the stress hormone. High levels of cortisol make you feel stressed out and anxious. By lowering cortisol levels, tulsi acts a natural anti-stress herb. Moreover, being an adaptogenic herb, tulsi contains anti-stress agents that help in soothing the nerves, fighting free radicals and regulating blood flow.

Skullcap

This herb is known for its abilities to relax tense muscles, reduce muscle spasms, calm nerves, and reduce headaches. Women will find skullcap tea to be very relieving because it's also known to bring down irritability associated with premenstrual syndrome.

Eat eggs for choline

Eat breakfast! Stop starving yourself. Many people with anxiety disorders skip breakfast. I recommend that people eat things like eggs, which are a satiating and filling protein, and are nature's top source of choline. Low levels of choline are associated with increased anxiety.

Exercise

Exercise is safe, good for the brain, and a powerful antidote to depression and anxiety, both immediately and in the long term. If you exercise on a regular basis, you'll have more self-esteem and feel healthier. One of the major causes of anxiety is worrying about illness and health, and that dissipates when you are fit. Even as little as 20 to 30 minutes of exercise can help alleviate stress and anxiety. From personal experience I can tell you that this is my favourite way to unwind!

Yoga

Hold your breath! Okay, let it out now. We're not recommending that you turn blue, but yoga breathing has been shown to be effective in lowering stress and anxiety. A classic yoga breathing technique is the 4-7-8. I do this myself and I love how it clears my brain of stressful thoughts.

One reason why it works is that you can't breathe deeply and be anxious at the same time. To do the 4-7-8 breath, exhale completely through your mouth, then inhale through your nose for a count of four. Hold your breath for a count of seven. Now let it out slowly through your mouth for a count of eight. Repeat at least twice a day.

Cozy up to fire with a tea

Ever wonder why you feel so relaxed after a spell in the sauna or a steam room? Heating up your body reduces muscle tension and anxiety, research has found. Sensations of warmth may alter neural circuits that control mood, including those that affect the neurotransmitter serotonin. Warming up may be one of the ways that exercise—not to mention curling up by a fire with a cozy cup of tea—boosts mood.

Whether lying on the beach in the midday sun on a Caribbean island, grabbing a few minutes in the sauna or spa after work, or sitting in a hot bath or Jacuzzi in the evening, we often associate feeling warm with a sense of relaxation and well-being.

Give yourself credit

Are you having anxious thoughts? Congratulations. You're aware of your emotional state, and that awareness is the first step in reducing anxiety.

Remember to give yourself credit for being aware that you are having anxious thoughts, and probably body changes. This is truly a skill of mindfulness that must be learned, and is essential in making the next steps of intervening through strategies such as positive self-talk, cognitive reframing, or the use of mindfulness or relaxation strategies.

Final thoughts

This world has been blessed with a lot of great choices for teas, herbal teas, and more, to help us fight the biggest battle in our personal world. Some may help you, some may not, but try to help yourself, every day, by drinking tea. I hope my story helps you in your fight against anxiety. Writing it down on paper really helped ease mine.

And don't forget that most of these herbs or teas can be found at your local loose-leaf tea store, health food store, or even in your own backyard. Many of these herbs grow in North America, and it is always a good idea to grow your own so that you can control the quality of the herb itself. Buy your seeds from a reputable source and buy organic tea if possible. Now relax, sit back, and have a cup of tea. Enjoy!

Yerba Maté:
The Healthy Energizer Brought to You by Nature's Synergy

Rosscoe Marks

I have used Yerba Maté for years while living in Bracebridge. I have shared this tea with many. When it was time to look for sponsors for The Anxiety Warrior Project, *I went through my cupboard and called the companies that I use. Rosscoe has been so supportive, I had to meet him and the sustainable company he works for in Winnipeg, Canada. I am so pleased that he was willing to share his passion for this type of tea.*

— Elke

There was a time when I drank coffee by the litre—forget cups!—and managed my stress levels with a most unhealthy smoking habit. I have to admit, I enjoyed the flavour and aroma of coffee and never imagined I'd start my day without it. Of course, I knew that smoking is a slow death and wanted to quit, but the stress of trying to quit caused me to want to smoke more.

After nearly two decades of bad habits, my life was a mess and I knew I had to do something. I was too anxious to sleep properly and completely dependent on coffee and cigarettes. I understood that my bad habits were symptoms of a bigger problem with the foundation of my life. My social relationships were unstable, and I was unhappy about everything.

Today, I have every reason to be thankful for the life I have. I no longer habitually drink coffee, and I have not smoked for years. The truth is, I couldn't do this alone. In the time of my desperate need, I made choices that led me to be surrounded by friends who have helped me understand that sustainable living requires sustainable human relationships. That sustainability is founded on a mutual recognition that as friends we need each other, and in our support for one another we realize in greater ways our purpose as human beings.

Early in my quest for a greater quality of life, I discovered yerba maté. It has replaced coffee for me, albeit in moderate quantities, as a consequence of having a more stable outlook on life. Maté consumption helped alleviate the withdrawal symptoms associated with cutting off a well-entrenched smoking habit. As a coffee replacement, maté provides the energy I need without the negative side effects of habitual coffee consumption. And, my discovery of this amazing beverage from South America, made from the yerba maté plant, landed me a job with a leading Canadian supplier of yerba maté, Maté Factor, where I learned more about the beverage's value and benefits.

Yerba maté—what it is and a brief history

Let's start with pronunciation. "Yerba" sounds as it is spelled; "maté" sounds like "mott ay."

The words "yerba maté" are anglicized from Spanish, Portuguese, and a South American indigenous language. They refer to a hot or cold beverage made from an infusion of the leaves of the yerba maté plant. The beverage is sometimes simply called maté.

Yerba maté—the plant

The yerba maté plant is actually an evergreen tree from the Aquifoliaceae family (which includes holly) that grows in the subtropical forests of South America; specifically, northern Argentina, Paraguay, Uruguay, and southern Brazil. The tree stands from six to eight metres tall, sometimes reaching as high as 15 metres.

There are many different species in the family: the Ilex genus having more than 550. In South America there are 280 species, 60 of which occur in southern Brazil. Only three species are used in the maté industry (I. angustifolia, I. amara, and I. paraguariensis, the most important). The maté plant, owing to the widespread genetic variety of the Ilex family, may have white or light purple stems and thick waxy leaves that may present dented or smooth edges.

History and culture

Long before Europeans arrived in South America, the indigenous people living in the heart of the continent understood the health benefits of yerba maté, and drank it for its gentle but powerful stimulating effect. To this day, it is customary for South Americans in the yerba maté growing region to gather in circles around a fire and drink maté from a common vessel, usually a hollowed out woody fruit called a gourd. The stimulating, mood-enhancing effects of yerba maté contribute to social interaction and conversation that are essential to sustainable living and human relationships.

When the Spanish and then the Portuguese arrived in the maté region of South America, they quickly recognized its commercial value. The Jesuits in northern Argentina were the first to cultivate yerba maté for commercial purposes. Though widespread use among European settlers became a source of anxiety for colonial authorities, over the centuries yerba maté became a cultural influence that served to colonize the Europeans into a new South American identity. Today, in a large part of South America, maté is more widely consumed than coffee.

Since the late 19th century, immigrant and expatriate migration has seen yerba maté spread to the Middle East and become an integral part of local cultures in that region. Yerba maté has been in North America for over 30 years. Today, while rising in popularity, it still remains widely unknown.

The energizing and health benefits of yerba maté

If you are familiar with maté, then you are familiar with the energizing effects of the beverage. If you believe that drinking maté reduces stress and anxiety, and has an uplifting effect on your mood, know that these benefits are not imagined. Centuries of use and modern research confirm this as reality. Yerba maté appears to be unique as an energizer, free of side effects common to drinking coffee, or black and green tea. Consuming maté late in the afternoon and early evening can enhance the quality of sleep.

More research is required to fully explain the unique energizing qualities of yerba maté. The secret appears locked in the synergistic relationship that the stimulating xanthine alkaloids, such as caffeine, theobromine, and theophylline, have with the vast array of active chemical constituents found in the plant.

Yes, there is a modest amount of caffeine in maté; similar levels as in an average cup of black and green tea, or a weak cup of coffee. However, consumer experience and modern research demonstrate that people who cannot drink coffee or tea due to caffeine intolerance do quite well enjoying a cup of maté. Researchers are unable to fully explain why this is the case, postulating only that the infusion of yerba maté in hot or cold water is a healthy energizer due to the natural synergy of its chemical constituents.

The health benefits of yerba maté are easier to understand than its energizing effects. Early research in the mid 1960s lauded the plant as having all the nutritive requirements for healthy human living. Subsequent research in later decades has not revealed another plant that surpasses yerba maté in nutritional value. On the antioxidant index, green tea is very close, but yerba maté appears to have active, nutritive chemicals not found in green tea.

It is reasonable to imagine that the vast nutritive spectrum found in yerba maté has everything to do with why the plant can be considered a healthy energizer. However, this subject is too vast for this article and suggestions for further reading appear at the end of this article.

Choosing the right yerba maté for you

Yerba maté comes in many variations, each with unique tastes and characteristics. Here's what I've learned in my time with Maté Factor.

Competing traditions define the form, quality, and consumption of yerba maté. In Argentina, Paraguay, and Uruguay it is common to cure fresh yerba maté by open fires. Heat is required to strip the leaves of protective enzymes that would otherwise hinder the drying process and speed up oxidization. Ancient methods are sometimes crude. Open fires imbue the dried maté with a smoky taste and turn the naturally green maté to various shades of brown. This process can cook the maté to a certain extent, which damages its nutritional value. Brazilian preferences favour little or no smoky flavour, and a greener maté. I prefer the Brazilian style because it preserves the life-giving nutrients and fresh green taste.

Consistent flavour is the product of great care and expertise in the harvesting and blending of the final product. There are minor variations in the presence of a slight bitterness due to the time of year the maté is harvested, and varying soil conditions. Cultivated yerba maté tends to have a stronger flavour than the wild plant, due to a greater percentage of stimulating xanthine alkaloids. Both wild and cultivated yerba maté are blended after the curing and drying process to ensure consistency in flavour, quality, and cut.

From the beginning, Maté Factor has been certified by international organic standards as a primary producer and food manufacturer. Organic standards ensure yerba maté is free of pesticides, herbicides, and every other toxic chemical common to conventional agriculture. The standards also complement care and diligence in upholding best practices in the cultivation, harvesting, processing, and production of yerba maté products. This commitment guarantees good stewardship of the natural environment, and consistent quality of the product for resale with the good health of the consumer in mind.

Wide product variety for the maté consumer

The products listed and described below are available in Canada through Maté Factor. Similar or additional products may be available from other suppliers. Please see the section "Suggested reading" for sources of detailed product descriptions, product availability, and contact information for Maté Factor.

The relatively mild and neutral flavour of fresh green yerba maté makes it an ideal base for flavourful blends of herbs and spices. At Maté Factor, certified organic whole spices and the freshest herbs are used as much as possible. Whole spices are milled as needed to ensure that the tea blends have the freshest taste. No flavourings are ever used.

Seven of nine blends have green yerba maté as a base. The other two have roasted maté. The roasting process alters the chemical constituents in the plant and dramatically alters the flavour. For people with a caffeine sensitivity, roasted maté might be too strong. It should be noted that green yerba maté blends have a lower percentage by weight, making the herb and spice blends ideal for people who cannot drink coffee or black and green tea due to a caffeine intolerance.

Here's a sampling of yerba maté products available in Canada:

✦ *Brazilian green*, a fresh green yerba maté from Brazil.

✦ *Extreme green*. Base: fresh green maté. Not for people with a caffeine intolerance. Green tea and guarana pack this tea with a caffeine punch that is as powerful as a strong cup of coffee, though still without the negative side effects associated with drinking coffee. The addition of eleuthero root, an adaptogen, caps the extreme in the green.

✦ *Cardamom chai.* Base: fresh green maté. This is a genuine chai blend made from whole spices sourced from around the world. It goes very well with milk and honey.

✦ *Lemon ginger.* Base: fresh green maté. Lemon myrtle and ginger are blended to make a delicious cup of tea. Popular in the winter, and soothing to sore throats.

✦ *Cinnamon rooibos.* Base: fresh green maté. Cinnamon from Asia mixes well with red rooibos from South Africa. People who enjoy cinnamon and rooibos will appreciate this blend.

✦ *Tropical sunrise.* Base: fresh green maté. Hibiscus, rosehips, lemon myrtle, lemongrass, and dried limes combine to present a tropical citrus beverage with a rich, red colour. This tea is superb served cold in summer heat.

✦ *Earl green.* Base: fresh green maté. Black tea complements the flavour of green maté. Blended with a measured dose of bergamot oil, this tea is a worthy variation of an old classic.

✦ *Green tea ginseng.* Base: fresh green maté. Maté Factor blends green tea with red panax ginseng and echinacea root and leaf to make this medicinal offering. This blend is very popular in cold and flu season. A note of caution for people sensitive to caffeine: this is a very stimulating blend. Use a little honey to cut the bitter flavour of the echinacea.

✦ *Dark roast.* Base: roasted maté. As noted above, roasted maté is not green maté. People with a caffeine intolerance should try this blend with caution. That said, roasted chicory and barley combine to make an absolutely delicious drink with added milk and honey. Many people have commented that this blend makes the ideal coffee replacement. While its taste and energizing qualities are similar to coffee, it is without the negative side effects associated with drinking coffee.

+ *Mocha mint.* Less than half of this blend by weight is roasted maté. Over half the blend is carob, which, combined with peppermint and roasted maté, make a pleasant dessert tea for everyone. Try it with milk and honey.

Yerba maté notes and tips

The following suggestions will help ensure you enjoy the benefits of yerba maté.

+ If you have a caffeine intolerance, use yerba maté tea products with caution.

+ Drink your water. Xanthine alkaloids are diuretics. Maté Factor recommends drinking a cup of water with every cup of yerba maté, whether roasted or green. This is in addition to the water we should normally drink.

+ Wet fresh green yerba maté with a little cold water before infusing in hot water. Doing this makes for a smoother drink. Follow steeping instructions on the package. Do not over-steep in hot water.

+ To make cold maté from a hot infusion, make the maté double strength and pour over ice at the end of the recommended steeping time.

+ Another method of making fresh green maté, hot or cold, is a cold steep. Add 250 grams (about one cup) of loose maté per four litres (about one US gallon) of cold water and refrigerate in a covered pot for six to eight hours. Strain out the loose tea before drinking it cold, or heating to the ideal drinking temperature for a hot beverage. This method makes the best maté you'll ever drink.

+ Add a dash of fresh lemon juice to a cup of cold, fresh green maté.

+ Never simmer or boil fresh green yerba maté. It will become very bitter.

Suggested reading

Wikipedia is an excellent source of information on both the yerba maté plant, and its history of use. Maté Factor, http://www.matefactor.ca, also provides valuable information on yerba maté.

You can also find a wealth of information available online that points to primary sources. Your local library, or university library will have additional resources to meet your level of interest.

Essential Oils for Anxiety

Chantelle Denstedt

Essential oils have been in my cupboard since I was a teenager. Along with health benefits, I enjoy the sensory pleasure that they provide. I had the good fortune of meeting Chantelle with whom I share a passion for essential oils.

— Elke

If you had asked me a year ago if I had ever suffered from anxiety, I would have said no. However, the more I learn about anxiety, the more I recognize the symptoms in myself and others. I believe we just push through life trying to deal with things, not listening to our bodies or recognizing certain symptoms. At least, this is how it has been for me.

If I were truthful with myself, I'd admit that my heart races. I get what feels like heart palpitations, and a decade ago I went so far as to have my heart tested, to only be told that, like many moms juggling children and a job, I was suffering from anxiety attacks. I realized that I just needed to find coping mechanisms to deal with the stress in my life, and the anxiety that came from this stress. Reading books, drinking tea, talking walks in nature, focused breathing, and alone time have been a few of the tools that I use to manage stress and anxiety, but then essential oils entered into my life, and these little oily gems soon became my passion.

I was first introduced to, and started using, essential oils in 2015. I have always had a strong belief in naturopathic and plant-based medicine. I believe in using the gifts provided to us by God (or Mother Nature), and resist taking modern medicine. Our bodies have a remarkable innate ability to heal themselves. The natural state of humans is health, not disease, and the body is equipped to fight a variety of illnesses and injuries that cause disease. Just look at the way a broken bone can mend, and a cut in our skin heals. Our bodies are amazing.

As I started to incorporate essential oils into my life, I become obsessed with learning more and researched as much as I could about how the oils work and affect our bodies. I also began to learn about environmental factors, and how they can have a negative impact on our lives, not only with our physical health but with our mental well-being as well.

Unfortunately, it is next to impossible to escape all the toxins present in our environment today. A number of these toxins are what are known as endocrine disrupters—chemicals that may interfere with the body's endocrine system and produce adverse developmental, reproductive, neurological, and immune effects in both humans and wildlife.

We can find these endocrine disrupters in many of our own household products and cleaning supplies. We know from pollution readings that there are harmful chemicals in the air that we breathe. However, studies show that the average North American home is more toxic and contains more harm to the human than being outdoors. According to the Huffington Post, the average women will apply 515 synthetic chemicals on her body daily.[1] However, we do have the control to change this and can start replacing all of our cleaning products, household products, and skin care products with natural plant-based and essential-oil-based products today, without too much effort and without "breaking the bank."

I personally can testify that the household products that I now make or use are just as effective, if not better than, the products I used to purchase. And I believe that my grandparents and great-grandparents would be pleased to see that I'm just going back to basics and using the same ingredients they used.

So what are essential oils?

Essential oils are powerful "Earth medicines" or concentrated extracts that are distilled from the bark, leaves, blooms, seeds, and roots of living plants, such as trees, shrubs, flowers, and herbs.

I like to think of essential oils as the plant's immune system. They are the most powerful part of the plant. They are its life blood. Just as our blood clots our cuts, oxygenates our cells and detoxifies our bodies, oils do the same for plants. They are the part of the plant that enables change.

Simply put, plants need some ability—some chemistry—to defend themselves from infections, damage, predators, and weather. The essential oil is the chemistry part of the plant that does this. For example, the essential oil of Frankincense comes from a tree (*Boswellia carterii* or *Boswellia sacara*) in Northern Africa. If the tree is scraped or cut, as it is during the distillation process, it produces sap to heal the wound and protect the tree. This oil is known to have anti-scarring properties that can provide support for our skin and immune system, just like it does for the tree.

Essential oils are extremely complex and can contain from 100 to 1,000 different natural chemical compounds. These chemical compounds protect the plant by helping it adapt to changes in the environment around it. It is these chemical compounds that enable individual oils to treat a variety of symptoms. The body uses the oil for what the body needs, so that the oil may have a different effect on each person.

In humans, these oils can provide support for every system in the body, including the skeletal, muscular, circulatory, and endocrine systems: they support our hormones and brain health, and are used extensively for emotional and spiritual support.

History

Essential oils have been around for centuries, dating back as far as biblical days, with more than 200 references to incense and ointments throughout the Bible. In fact, the baby Jesus was given frankincense and myrrh as gifts. Ancient texts and historical and archaeological evidence, including Egyptian hieroglyphs, Chinese manuscripts, Greek physicians' records, and biblical references, suggest that essential oils have been an integral part of health and wellness for centuries.[2]

So how do essential oils help with anxiety?

Our sense of smell is the only one of the five senses directly tied to the limbic area of the brain, which is considered the emotional control centre. When essential oils are inhaled, they go directly to our brain. Because the limbic system is connected to the parts of the brain that control heart rate, blood pressure, breathing, memory, stress levels, and hormone balance, therapeutic-grade essential oils can have unbelievable psychological effects. Their use is recommended by institutes such as the Mayo Clinic[3] and the National Cancer Institute.[4] Numerous studies can be found in "Pubmed,"[5] the U.S. National Library of Medicine's database of scientific research. It lists over 15,000 studies on the use and benefits of essential oils.

Aromatherapy is a healing technique that uses essential oils by tapping into the powerful relationship between smell and the brain. Our sense of smell is quite powerful. Do you ever smell something and are transported back to an event in time? What does the smell of a pine tree remind you of? Or a campfire? Or the smell after a spring shower? So many smells can trigger memories that transport me back to my childhood.

As noted above, scent receptors in the nose send chemical messages to the limbic system, by way of the olfactory nerve. The limbic system is the part of the brain that deals with basic emotions like anger and fear, happiness and joy, and emotional trauma, anxiety, stress, and depression. It's our sense of smell that allows essential oils to directly combat negative emotions.

How to incorporate them into your life

How can you use oils to help relieve anxiety? Diffuse the oil in your home. Apply it topically to your skin, using a carrier oil such as olive oil, coconut oil, or jojoba oil to dilute it. Carry diluted oil in a glass roller bottle and apply as needed, or wear it on porous jewellery such as a lava rock.

If you plan to add essential oils to your toolkit, use a therapeutic grade, unadulterated essential oil only. Avoid oils that have been extracted with a chemical solvent, or diluted with a synthetic. You will not reap the health benefits of the essential oil, and the solvents and synthetics could hurt you. Unfortunately, manufacturers can label an essential oil as pure or therapeutic grade as long as 5 percent of the contents of the bottle contain pure oil. That means the other 95 percent can be anything else.

The U.S. Toxic Substance Control Act[6] of 1976 grandfathered an estimated 65,000 to 100,000 chemicals still on the market today, which means these chemicals have not had any safety testing and we know very little about their effects. Further, under the act manufacturers are not required to list product ingredients, toxic or otherwise, if the item is not consumable. And these manufacturers are protected by trade secret laws that allow them to keep their ingredients a secret. Many of these ingredients are hidden under the word "fragrance."

How do you know if the oil is pure?

When it comes right down to it, you need to trust the company that you are purchasing from. It is "Unthinkable that women and men would knowingly inflect such exposures on their infants, children and themselves if products routinely used were labeled with explicit warning of cancer risks," says Dr. Samuel Epstein, chairman of the Cancer Prevention Coalition, professor emeritus of Occupational and Environmental Medicine at the University of Illinois, School of Public Health at Chicago, and a leading international authority on toxicology and the carcinogenic effects of contaminants in consumer products.

What to look for when purchasing essential oils

When buying an essential oil, ensure that the company:

- ✦ Has expertise in the distillation process and innovative distillation equipment.

- ✦ Has published essential oils research in scientific journals, particularly surrounding distillation procedures.

- ✦ Owns their own farms/land, or at a minimum is involved in the farming and cultivation process.

- ✦ Ensures that the land is free of fertilizers and pesticides.

- ✦ Has in-house laboratories to test oils for purity, and verifies the purity with their own laboratories, as well as with third-party testing facilities.

- ✦ Has qualified staff who understand the testing methods and have experience reading analyses.

You can find much of this information on company websites.

Best oils for anxiety

So now that you understand a bit more about essential oils, how they work, and how you can use them, which ones should you start with? There are so many, but I'm going to share five of my favourites.

+ *Lavender* is probably one of the most popular oils, but because of its popularity many lavender oils available for purchase are often adulterated with a hybrid lavender called lavendin, or with synthetic fragrance chemicals like ethyl vanillin. Therapeutic lavender essential oils offer the following benefits:

    ✧ calms, relaxes, and balances us both physically and emotionally.

    ✧ restores the nervous system.

    ✧ helps inner peace, and reduces restlessness, irritability, and panic attacks.

    ✧ promotes a good night's sleep.

Anxiety and stress can overstimulate a person trying to settle down for the night. Worries and fears cause tension that keeps a person awake, yet sleep is so important to our overall well-being. Sleep is rejuvenating. Lavender can help calm the body and prepare it for a good night's rest.

University of Miami researchers found that inhalation of lavender oil fragrance increased beta waves in the brain, suggesting heightened relaxation. It also reduced depression and improved cognitive performance (Diego MA, et el., 1998). A 2001 Osaka Kyoiku University study found that lavender reduced mental stress and increased alertness (Motomura, 2001).[7]

Diffuse three to four drops of lavender in your diffuser, and/or apply lavender directly to the bottom of your big toe.

+ *Frankincense.* If I were allowed to have only one oil, I would choose frankincense. This is the essential oil that got me interested in the study of essential oils. Frankincense is considered a holy anointing oil in the

Middle East, and has been used in religious ceremonies for thousands of years. According to the Ebers Papyrus, a 3,700-year-old Egyptian list of prescriptions and recipes, frankincense was "Used to treat every illness know to man."[8] It was valued more than gold during ancient times, and only those with great wealth and abundance possessed it. Frankincense is mentioned in the Ebers Papyrus (16th century B.C.) in 877 prescriptions and recipes.

As recommended by Dr. Josh Axe, a certified doctor of natural medicine, doctor of chiropractic, and a clinical nutritionist in Nashville, frankincense is probably the best oil for neurological support. It helps with the function of the central nervous system in particular.

Whether it's helping with clarity of thinking, or balancing the emotions, frankincense has a lot of benefits to offer. Apply two to three drops of frankincense with a carrier oil to the back of your neck when feeling stressed. Diffuse a few drops at bedtime to help slow down your breathing and release nervous tension and anxiety.

✦ *Cedarwood. Cedrus atlantica* is the species most closely related to the biblical Cedar of Lebanon. It is believed to stimulate the limbic region of the brain (the centre of emotions) and the pineal gland, which releases melatonin. It is also recognized for its calming and purifying properties. While lavender helps prepare and relax me for a good night's sleep, I find that cedarwood gives me the deep sleep that I so need.

✦ *Vetiver* is used for Attention Deficit Hyperactivity Disorder (ADHD), anxiety, and depression (including postpartum), and to aid sleep. It is believed to be psychologically grounding, calming, tranquil, and stabilizing, and helps us cope with stress and recover from emotional trauma. A nervous system tonic, it decreases jitteriness and hypersensitivity, and is useful in panic attacks and shock. A number of my colleagues use vetiver with their young children if they have anxiety about going to school and being separated from their parents.

+ *Chamomile* is a relaxant that can help with insomnia. It is believed to soothe and clear the mind, dispel anger, and help release emotions linked to the past. An exploratory study[9] conducted at the University of Pennsylvania School of Medicine on the antidepressant activity in chamomile found that this essential oil "May provide clinically meaningful antidepressant activity that occurs in addition to its previously observed anxiolytic activity."

More research findings

In a 2014 study by the American College of Healthcare Sciences, 58 hospice patients were given hand massages once a day for one week with an essential oil blend in 1.5 percent dilution with sweet almond oil. The blend consisted of equal ratios of bergamot, frankincense, and lavender. All patients reported less pain and depression, concluding that aromatherapy massage with this blend is more effective for pain and depression management than massage alone.

Try using an essential oil today

Essential oils are commonly used with a diffuser. If you do not have one, you can use the following recipe to reap the benefits. Ensure that you are using a pure, unadulterated essential oil.

Ingredients: three drops of lavender and five millilitres (about one teaspoon) of fractionated coconut oil or almond oil.

Blend the oils in your palm and rub onto your neck for natural relief. You may also rub the mix onto to the bottoms of your feet, specifically the bottom of your big toes. Perfect for anytime, or just before bed.

Animals and essential oils

Not only do essential oils benefit humans, they can benefit our furry four-legged friends as well. Studies have proven that our pets help us with our anxiety. Animals sense our emotions, often through smell. However, animals suffer from anxiety as well.

Help your furry companions out by ditching animal products that contain harmful ingredients, especially "fragrance." There are essential oil and oil blends you can create that are effective for calming dogs that have separation anxiety, noise anxiety, or fear of new places and people. Here's one example:

Ingredients

15 ml (about ½ oz.) base oil (e.g., olive oil, sweet almond, or jojoba oil)

three drops valerian oil

three drops lavender oil

two drops of clary sage oil

two drops of sweet marjoram oil

To apply the oils topically, rub two to three drops of the essential oil blend between your hands and apply to the edge of your dog's ears, between the toes, on inner thighs, or "armpits." Lavender is another good oil to use for anxiety.

Conclusion

If you were to ask me what is the one thing that you could do today, I would beg you to ditch your scented candles and fragrances. I have. Some research suggests a possible link between certain health effects and chemicals used in these and other scented products, such as aerosols, plug-ins, gels, and incense sticks. Why take the chance? If you do not introduce essential oils into your house, at least start ridding your household of the unnecessary "fresheners" and "fragrances," and note how you start to feel.

Three Favourite Recipes

Foaming liquid hand soap
Ironically, I never liked foaming hand soap until I started making my own.

1.   Reuse or purchase a foaming hand-soap bottle.

2. Fill it approximately three-quarters full with water.*

3. Add 30 ml (about two tbsp.) Castile soap. (I use Dr. Bronner's, which can be purchased from any health food store, or health section of the grocery store. You'll soon find that Dr. Bronner's will become a new staple in your home.)

4. Add 5 ml (about one tsp.) fractionated coconut oil.

5. Add 10 drops of your favourite essential oil(s) (lavender, orange, peppermint, and lemon for the extra-clean smell. "Thieves" is an essential oil blend** proprietary to Young Living, that is helpful in the winter time to ward off colds. The blend is inspired by the legend of 15th-century French thieves who formulated a special aromatic combination of clove, rosemary, and other botanicals. It is an amazing blend of highly antiviral, antiseptic, antibacterial and anti-infectious essential oils.

6. Slowly top up with a bit more water, leaving room for foam at the top.

* *Always add water first. If you add the soap before the water, you're bound to have a foaming mess.*

** *Personally, I am now spoiled as I purchase the Thieves Household Cleaner. It is an amazing strong concentrate (one capful to two or three cups of water). It makes everything. I use it for my general cleaning, mirrors, dishwasher detergent, hardwood floors, stainless steel appliances, and furniture. Find out more:* www.youngliving.com/en_US/products/thieves-household-cleaner

Stainless steel appliance cleaner

Ingredients

14 ml (about one tbsp.) olive oil

14 ml (about one tbsp.) white vinegar

Directions

1. Add the olive oil to a soft cloth and rub the appliance's surface to get rid of smudges.

2. Fold cloth, add vinegar, and wipe down again.

3. With a dry side of the cloth, wipe again.

All-purpose surface cleaner

Ingredients

28 ml (about six oz.) white vinegar

28 ml (about six oz.) distilled water

10 drops lemon essential oil

12 drops lavender essential oil

Directions

Mix together in a 340 ml (about 12 oz.) spray bottle (preferably glass). Shake before each use. Use on toilets, tubs, sinks, counter tops, and walls. Wipe clean with a dry soft cloth or rag.

Additional resources:

Vivian C. Pun, Justin Manjourides, and Helen Suh, "Association of Ambient Air Pollution with Depressive and Anxiety Symptoms in Older Adults: Results from the NSHAP Study," Environmental Health Perspectives, 125:342-348: Department of Health Sciences, Northeastern University, Boston, MA, March 2017
https://ehp.niehs.nih.gov/ehp494/
"The Top 7 Essential Oils for Anxiety," by Dr. Josh Axe, January 2017.
https://draxe.com/about-dr-josh-axe/
https://draxe.com/what-is-frankincense/
https://draxe.com/essential-oils-for-anxiety/
"Dirty Dozen Endocrine Disruptors: 12 Hormone-Altering Chemicals and How to Avoid Them," Environmental Working Group, October 2013.
http://www.ewg.org/research/dirty-dozen-list-endocrine-disruptors

Notes

1 Michelle Persad, "The Average Woman Puts 515 Synthetic Chemicals on Her Body Every Day Without Knowing," *The Huffington Post*, March 7, 2016. http://www.huffingtonpost.ca/entry/synthetic-chemicals-skincare_us_56d8ad09e4b0000de403d995

2 Dr. Scott A. Johnson, *Surviving When Modern Medicine Fails: A Definitive Guide to Essential Oils That Could Save Your Life During a Crisis*, Createspace.

3 Brent A. Bauer, M.D., "What are the benefits of aromatherapy," Mayo Clinic, May 24, 2017. http://www.mayoclinic.org/healthy-lifestyle/consumer-health/expert-answers/aromatherapy/faq-20058566

4 "Aromatherapy and Essential Oils (PDQ®) - Patient Version," National Cancer Institute at the National Institutes of Health, U.S. Department of Health and Human Services, June 9, 2017. https://www.cancer.gov/about-cancer/treatment/cam/patient/aromatherapy-pdq

5 U.S. National Library of Medicine, National Institutes of Health, U.S. Department of Health and Human Services, 2018. https://www.ncbi.nlm.nih.gov/pubmed/?term=essential+oils

6 Toxic Substances Control Act (TSCA) and Federal Facilities, United States Environmental Protection Agency, January 19, 2017. https://www.epa.gov/enforcement/toxic-substances-control-act-tsca-and-federal-facilities

7 *Essential Oils Desk Reference, 6th Edition*, compiled by Life Science Publishing, 2014. http://www.ewg.org/research/dirty-dozen-list-endocrine-disruptors

8 *Essential Oils Desk Reference*, sixth edition compiled by Life Science Publishing, pg. 101 "'Used to treat every conceivable ill known to man,' frankincense was valued more than gold during ancient times, and only those with great wealth and abundance possessed it. It is mentioned in one of the oldest known medical records, *Ebers Papyrus* (dating from 16 century BC), an ancient Egyptian list of 877 prescriptions and recipes.'

9 J.D. Amsterdam, J.Shults, I. Soeller, J.J. Mao, K. Rockwell, and A.B. Newberg, "Chamomile (Matricaria recutita) may provide antidepressant activity in anxious, depressed humans: an exploratory study." University of Pennsylvania School of Medicine, September-October 2012. https://www.ncbi.nlm.nih.gov/pubmed/22894890.

The Sacred Tree

Susan O'Connell

I met Susan outside the Human Rights Museum in Winnipeg, Canada, after our IEATA conference this fall. We quickly realized we related on so many levels and I learned that ecotherapy is her passion. If I could I would spend all hours in nature. It is there I fill my cup, my soul. Susan is a gifted heartfelt professor, facilitator and writer sharing with us a way to reconnect to our Earth.

— Elke

Those who dwell among the beauties and mysteries of the Earth are never alone or weary of life... Those who contemplate the beauty of the Earth find reserves of strength that will endure as long as life lasts.
— Rachel Carson

This chapter explores our relationship with the natural world, and how our way of being in nature informs our sense of well-being and belonging. Cultivating a relationship with the natural world by bringing our relationship more fully into conscious awareness through engagement with nature opens our heart and invites us to care for the Earth. We also respond to the destruction of beloved neighbourhood and global habitats, and the loss of ecosystems and the wild ones who live there. Respect for the natural world and a reciprocal relationship with nature are essential ingredients in quality of life for all beings and our shared future.

This chapter is written through a lens of ecopsychology, which questions our illusion of separation from the natural world, and studies how this perspective, along with a physical distance from nature, influence our quality of life and the well-being of our Earth home.

There is much historical basis and scholarship surrounding the field of ecopsychology. In this short chapter, I will only touch on this briefly, and attempt to convey key points as they relate to well-being, particularly in the areas of grief, anxiety, feelings of helplessness, and what is often termed ecoanxiety. Wiktionary defines ecoanxiety as "anxiety about damage to the ecosystem." However, in this chapter we will also consider how we are impacted through a constricted relationship with the natural world and the anxiety this might cause.

In this writing, you will find simple experiential practices that offer a path towards cultivating a relationship with the more-than-human world, while fostering our unique ways of knowing beyond the intellect. I invite you to experiment and see for yourself how they inform you over time. When I engage in these types of contemplative practices in nature, they slow me down and enable me to be present. This offers me understanding in a new way; I begin to see things I hadn't noticed before. I begin to sense my deep connection and belonging to the human and the more than human world.

Deepening roots

If we surrendered to Earth's intelligence
we could rise up rooted, like trees.
— Rainer Maria Rilke

I was born and in raised in a small village high on the cliffs above the Pacific Ocean where the landscape formed a bay. When I was growing up, children were encouraged to be outdoors a good part of the day and into the evening. We were left alone in a blossoming natural world with our imaginations and our fantasies. And, even as I had many siblings, I found joy being alone in nature in active exploration or quiet reverie.

I recognize that through my early immersion in nature I first experienced an integration of body, mind, spirit, and heart, leaving me feeling connected to all life. I can best describe this as being fully awake and present in the world as she was at any given time, be that beautiful and serene, or wild and frightening. Most importantly, I was engaged in a relationship with an animate world inclusive of the wild beings who lived there: the wind, waves and the sea, the trees that lined my street, the birds that sang full throated from their perches, the green hills filled with mustard plants, and the white stars who unveiled their faces in the night sky. All these and more settled deeply into my heart and psyche, and I felt woven into the natural world.

Both of my parents were adult children of alcoholics and they brought their own unresolved issues into their marriage and family life. This resulted in inconsistent and inadequate parenting at times, which left me feeling uncertain and anxious about how I belonged. I experienced feelings of unworthiness. These feelings were painful, and limited my sense of security. One saving grace for me was that my parents were both creative individuals who loved nature. The natural and open spaces we frequented as a family were key ingredients in my resilience, and my ability to walk with my anxiety.

My early relationship with the natural world offered mitigating and enriching soil for imagination, creative energy, and solace. This Earth connection presented me with an opportunity as a child to provide offerings such as love, gratitude, compassion, and care even as I was the recipient of beauty and life lessons. The reciprocity in this relationship taught me much about how to be within myself, in relationship, and in the world. I am grateful that my parents provided frequent nature experiences, and for nature's role in my overall development.

When I entered the educational system as a child, I experienced what I have come to understand as a soul loss, in the way of feeling split off from my authentic self. I remember sitting in the hard-seated classroom for hours memorizing information that seemed abstracted from life, while glancing longingly through a window at the blue sea beyond a green field. From my school desk, I could hear the crashing of the ocean waves and the call of the seagulls, and smell the salt air. They seemed to be inviting me to join them, and I felt a strong pull to return to the natural world that was often painful. As I left school each day, running towards a grove of nearby trees with my brother, I experienced such a sense of happiness in sharp contrast to my six hours of non-experiential education. Over time, I learned to be in the school system as it was. However, part of my joy and aliveness was diminished through this social adjustment, which created an opening for further anxiety. I don't think my experience is unique, and I believe this anxiety can be mitigated by offering children more experiential and outdoor education.

As I grew into a young woman with a career and child of my own, the quality time I could spend in nature shrank. I don't think this is atypical for many of us in our busy world. But, here too, I experienced longing, sorrow, and a sense of loss. I did spend time in nature, but most often it was a visit rather than a way of being: the former offered temporary solace, while the latter offered foundational and ongoing relationship gifts.

To mitigate this sense of loss, a part of me compensated by becoming numb. The trouble with psychic numbing is that we can't just numb the painful aspects of our lives, rather we numb across the entire spectrum of feeling, including joy. In my case, this contributed to a dulling of life energy and movement away from my authentic self, which led me deeper into an experience of low-level anxiety. I did not recognize at that time the cause and effect.

Experiential #1: Remembrance—your nature story (15 minutes or more)

Find a quiet place where you feel safe and won't be disturbed, preferably in nature. Feel your feet on the ground where you are sitting or standing. Relax, close your eyes, and breathe deeply and slowly for a few minutes. Begin to remember times you have spent in the natural world; this could be as a child, as an adult in your garden, a walk you take nearby, or a time on vacation. As the scenes move through your mind's eye, settle on just one memory for this session.

Deepen into your memory. What sounds do you remember? What smells were present? What part of nature attracted your eye? Were there things you touched, and if so what was the texture? What is your memory of your overall sense of the experience? Just be fully present to the memory of your time in nature. Spend at least 15 minutes with this memory.

When you open your eyes, explore how your body feels. What is your experience of being present with a memory of a time in nature?

Journal your response or write a poem or use art-making materials to create a response.

Note: If you are unable to move outdoors for any of the experientials, please sit by a window that looks towards the outside or locate a nature video (e.g., YouTube), which provides nature images and sounds to immerse yourself in this for the time frame.

Tree bark

We inter-breathe with the rain forests,
We drink from the oceans.
They are part of our body.
—Thich Nhat Hanh

Ecopsychologists believe there is a direct and inseparable connection between our sense of well-being and the world around us. Yet, traditional psychology has been slow to recognize this, and rarely includes discussion about our feelings surrounding the natural world, our sense of place, or how the landscape around us influences our well-being.

Scofield and Margulis (2012) state that, "Traditional psychologies often overlook a major source of chronic psychological pain—the disconnect of modern humans from the Earth's biosphere" (p. 219). Davis (1998) explains the impact of our separation from nature in this way:

> "There is a deeply bonded and reciprocal communion between humans and nature. The denial of this bond is a source of suffering both for the physical environment and for the human psyche, and the realization of the connection between humans and nature is healing for both." (p. 6)

One of the consequences of this movement away from nature has been our loss of daily integrated connection to nature's beauty and wisdom. In today's world, we may place priority on activities other than being in the natural world. We have forgotten, or quickly forget, encounters with the natural world that open our heart and ease the stress of our lifestyle. We forget the way nature's beauty and wildness inform us of our own beauty and wildness. In our distance from nature, we may forget the sense of gratitude we experience when emerging from a walk taken deep within the forest, or the sense of awe when we stand near a mountain peak laden with snow on a blue sky'd day.

Our feelings of grief and anxiety over the loss of connection with natural areas makes sense when we remember we evolved in animal bodies closely connected to and interdependent with a natural world that was understood to be alive and infused with spirit and voice. It is only recently in the evolutionary cycle that we began spending most of our days indoors rather than outdoors.

With the advent of technological tools, we are further disconnected from the allure of nature, which may have a softer voice in contrast to the addictive pull of technology. Of course, there are many life-giving benefits of technology; however, much of our free time, and our children's free time, is now spent with technology rather than in the sensual world around us. When our time in nature is absent or constricted, we lose a significant way of relationship and understanding about our kinship with all beings. We might notice this as we experience our sense of belonging within the natural world slipping away. The natural world feels like a stranger and our inclination to approach her takes effort. Our memories of happy and even transformative times in the natural world grow dim through lack of attention, which may result in feeling less love for Earth and less compassion for the wild ones who live nearby. When we feel disconnection from the natural world, we may notice feelings of anxiety, separation, or alienation and not quite know from where they arise.

The hope here resides in the knowledge that early childhood experiences in nature have a deep impact on us (*Louv, 2008*). Throughout our lives, we may hear the Earth's call, even when we are far removed from our experiences in nature. If we do hear that call, it is important to answer it by moving our body into a green area near home. This small "yes" movement may invite deeper memories of being in nature that offer nourishment, and act as an opening to cultivating a deeper relationship with nature. And, our willingness to share the gifts of the Earth with our children is very important and has consequences now, and for decades to come.

In my own experience, a way of being that is open to the more-than-human world acts as an opening to a wider and deeper perception, self-awareness, and mind/body/spirit integration. When I attend to Earth's rhythms and seasonal cycles, I encounter depths within myself, both hopes and dreads, of which I was not consciously aware. A quiet or contemplative approach to nature not only opens our powers of somatic and sensory intelligence, but invites our imagination and intuition to take the lead for a time, rather than the intellectual rational mind. This can be a delicious experience in our sensory-deprived world of technology, and our response may surprise us. We may become attuned to the creative energy of nature and feel inspired to express our own creativity. Other feelings that might arise through being in nature include gratitude, wonder, awe, or reverence, and there may also be uncomfortable feelings such as uncertainty, anxiety, longing, or grief regarding our recognition of the destruction of our beautiful Earth.

Experiential #2: Sensual awareness/intelligence (30 minutes)

This exercise will ask you to pay close attention to your senses using technology in contrast to your senses in being within the natural world. Plan to spend at least 15 minutes with each activity (for a total of 30 minutes) and then a time for journaling after each immersion.

First, find a safe and quite place in nature; this could be in your garden, a community garden, a park, wilderness area, the seashore, etc. Sit quietly. Breathe deeply and become present to all that surrounds you. Open your senses one by one by noticing smells, sounds, textures, and what is visible to you. Just be present to nature. When you feel complete, write in your journal about your experience.

How did this experience inform you? What did your focus shift towards? How connected did you feel towards your body? The body of Earth? Your mind? Your spirit?

Second, for 15 minutes use social media, TV, or another technology you regularly use. At the end of this session, write about your experience and what you felt.

Again, attend to how this experience informed you. How did your focus shift? How connected did you feel towards your body? The body of Earth? Your spirit? Where was the focus of your awareness (mind, body)?

Finally, review the two experiences and your journal notes. Note any similarities or differences. In particular, note how time in nature and with technology influenced your sense of discomfort or anxiety and your connection to your body and the body of Earth.

Welcoming branches

> Go back and take care of yourself. Your body
> needs you, your feelings need you. Your suffering,
> your blocks of pain need you. Your deepest
> desire needs you to acknowledge it.
> Go home and be there for these things...
> Do everything in mindfulness so you
> can really be there, so you can love
>
> *Thich Nhat Hanh (2007, p. 82)*

Many of us have learned through our cultural belief system that Earth is an inanimate place that serves us by providing resources for our use and disposal. This is in sharp contrast to many Indigenous (or non-western) cultures who understand Earth as a living spirited being; an ecosystem with presence and voice, one which supports many forms of life including human life (Abrams, 1996, Harding, 2006). Still, for many of us, especially those who are sensitive or have experienced connection with the natural world, we recognize the wonderful diversity of life around us, and may experience sorrow as we recognize familiar and beautiful wild places destroyed.

When we read or hear about the ongoing destruction of the natural world around us—species becoming extinct, water and air pollution, chemicals in our foods—we might encounter feelings of anger, anxiety, sorrow, grief and even a sense of being overwhelmed. These emotions are natural responses when we witness death and decay, and yet we may not connect this grief and sorrow with our ongoing witness of the distress and decline of animal and plant species, forests, water and air quality, and habitats of beauty. My experience is that bringing awareness to these issues and to the feelings evoked, while painful, also gives us the opportunity to take action, which mitigates our sense of helplessness.

Even as these are normal responses to such information, being open to the feelings that arise can be painful. This is particularly so for sensitive people who may already be experiencing anxiety. Our inclination when facing uncomfortable feelings might have us moving away from them; perhaps we distract ourselves or become numb so that we won't feel the pain. Buzzell and Chailquist (2009) write,

The problem of our day is an inner deadening, an increasingly deployed defence against the stresses of loving in an overbuilt industrialized civilization saturated by intrusive advertising and media, unregulated toxic chemicals, unhealthy food, parasitic business practices, time-stressed living... No wonder many of us disconnect, and resort to medication or other addictions in an attempt to temporarily drown out external hostilities. (p. 19)

There are certainly times when it is appropriate to shield our energy from too much disturbing information. Being mindful of how and what we ingest by way of news and information becomes increasingly important for us as individuals, and if we are parents of young children. We are cultivating self-compassion when we monitor and screen how many images or news reports we invite into our psyche, especially when we feel depleted. It is important to maintain balance by also considering the many ways people are responding with energy, generosity, and heart throughout the world. These responses may not be as visible to us in the news reporting, but they do exist (I have listed some resources at the end of the chapter). And, finally, we must pay attention to the signals that indicate it is an appropriate time to seek a companion or professional to help us in our journey through the challenges we face in today's world. To recognize and seek assistance is a sign of wisdom.

One concern when we distract or numb ourselves to avoid uncomfortable feelings is that we may miss an opportunity for self-understanding and growth; we may constrict our capacity to find meaning and integration through standing with the total of who we are. If we are able to befriend our deepest feelings, what might we learn? The difficult feelings we encounter through our disconnection with nature may offer us a path of counter practice, one in which we intentionally bring ourselves into a deeper connection with our feelings, and with nature. Joanna Macy (2003) explains that when we understand the depth of our sorrow we also notice the depth of our capacity to love, and our belonging to the world. She writes that this awareness is a source "from which comes the power to endure hardship and to act for the well-being of all" (p. 160). Through our presence and self-reflection, we may learn to hold many emotions while cultivating empathy and compassion for the human and more-than-human world.

In my teaching, the students explore these issues within the safety and community of a group. Each arrive with their own understanding of life through their cultural belief systems and their lived experience. Each have strengths in an area that others lack, so each student has a unique contribution that offers the group insight into how to consciously walk in the world with their feelings, and how to mentor others in their growth. These types of community explorations invite us to consider aspects of our individual and collective belief systems, and how they might contribute to the destruction of our Earth habitat that sustains us.

If we do choose to explore the labyrinth of grief or sorrow regarding the Earth's health, we encounter the very heart of an experience shared by many. This is a global issue and if we can speak with others in our home and community, we find we are not alone; many share our anxiety over the state of the world. However, through these engagements, we may also find nourishing depths of communication and an opening of understanding. When we allow ourselves to be touched by what we encounter, even when we do not have the power to change it, we may begin to engage in greater compassion and care of ourselves, all beings, and the Earth.

Green sunlit leaves

> Humankind has not woven the web of life. We are but one thread within it. Whatever we do to the web, we do to ourselves. All things are bound together. All things are connected.
> — Chief Seattle (in Ingerman, 2000, p. 131)

One antidote to ecoanxiety available to most of us is to move into a new way of being with the natural world. When we courageously step into cultivating a relationship with nature, a way of being mindful and open to all beings, we begin to notice the rich aliveness available to us. (Sewell, 2012). We begin to realize that there are numerous animate beings present who are observing us even as we observe them. This has always been so, but in our busyness we have not developed the eyes and heart to see them. We begin to see the world around us as she is: as a living being, a vibrant interconnected ecosystem within which human life is only a small interwoven part. As we continue to spend time in nature, we may find ourselves in kinship with the more than human world, unified and not separate. We may recognize through our connection to the world that we are embedded within a blossoming Earth and also dependent upon her. We may begin to value our ways of knowing beyond the intellectual, and begin to recognize the voices from Earth. Abrams (1996) says poetically:

> As we return to our senses, we gradually discover our sensory perceptions to be simply one part of a vast, interpenetrating web work of perceptions and sensations borne by countless other bodies—supported, that is, not just by ourselves, but by icy streams tumbling down granitic slopes, by owl wings and lichens, and by the unseen, imperturbable wind. (p. 65)

Experiential #3: Contemplation in nature; opening to all beings (20 minutes)

Find a safe and quiet place where you can walk in nature. Get comfortable and bring your attention to the world around you. For this exercise, please walk slowly and in silence.

As you begin, open yourself to the world around you. Recognize and give attention to each of your senses in turn and how they respond to the natural world: the sight, the sounds, the smells, and the textures. Stop whenever you wish to really be present to the world around you.

Just be gently aware of all that is present as you continue your time in nature.

When you have completed the walk, consider your quality of presence in nature. How did your body respond? What arose for you? Is there an invitation for you?

One benefit of walking or sitting in nature is that our body may respond to the Earth with a grounded feeling, which can be beneficial when anxiety is present. Contemplative walking practices are included in my daily life, and I hope you can integrate them into yours as well.

Blossoms and fruit

To see a World in a Grain of Sand
And a Heaven in a Wild Flower
Hold Infinity in the palm of your hand
And Eternity in an hour

— William Blake

One hidden gem in reconnecting with nature is that we may develop a relationship that opens our heart. Having love for another is when we most often act in their behalf. It is through an ongoing relationship with the natural world that we are most often inspired to care for the Earth and all beings (Harding, 1997, Macy 2003). As we begin to take actions to care for the Earth, no matter how small we may think our work is, we loosen the grip of helplessness and anxiety. This can ease our feelings of alienation and increase our empowerment and sense of belonging. We are now engaging in a reciprocal relationship with our habitat, the Earth, by taking action in service of life. In this case, life means our self, the human family, the Earth, sky, sea and beyond, all beings embedded within the body of Earth, and the children of future generations. As our hearts open through our experience within nature and nature care, we may begin to find new ways to contribute to the well-being of Earth, and, through our example, others witness a different way to be in the world. This is one form of activism at the grassroots level, and quite powerful.

Experiential #4: Choosing one sustainable action in care of the Earth

Please look at the list below. Consider the busyness of your schedule and life, and choose one action that you can absorb on a daily or weekly basis (in addition to your walks or time spent in nature). The key here is not how big the contribution is, rather that it be sustainable in an ongoing way. It is not helpful to choose something time consuming if it is wearing and unsustainable. Please start small. You can add on later if you wish. There are many things you may already be doing in care of the Earth, and I thank you. You may also have your own idea about how to take action that is not listed, due to space.

Sustainable actions in care of Earth

a) Working in your home or community

✦ Garden quietly in your yard or a nearby community garden.

✦ Clean a park in your community.

✦ Capture gray water from your shower and use it to water outside plants.

✦ Buy and use canvas bags for purchases.

✦ Ride your bike, carpool, or walk to work.

✦ Learn about the wildlife in your neighbourhood.

✦ Consider planting native plants around your area.

✦ Learn where organic farms are in your area and frequent them.

✦ Learn about pesticides and where they are used nearby.

✦ Create an organic garden or a community garden.

✦ Use creative expression to support the Earth.

✦ Create a collage with fallen natural materials (not picked).

b) Working with children or young adults

✦ Teach a younger person about being in a relationship with nature.

✦ Teach a younger person about interconnection and ecosystems.

✦ Garden with a child. Walk in nature with a child; skip, perhaps.

✦ Create a nature collage together on the ground.

✦ Teach a child bird calls or plant names. Splash in the water with a child.

c) *Working with a housebound elderly person (your relative, a neighbour or nursing home resident)*

✦ Bring flowers, and if appropriate ask them about a place they love.

✦ Create a photo slide show or bring photographs of nature to share.

✦ Bring a pet to visit.

✦ If they are able, sit with them outside or near a window or take them on a drive to a natural area.

✦ Provide a nature CD or video.

✦ Provide a poster of a beautiful nature scene to hang near them.

✦ Garden with them.

If they are in a nursing facility ask the director to create a garden that clients can go to and even work in, if they are able.

d) *Volunteerism and/or activism*

✦ Volunteer with an environmental group.

✦ Volunteer with a university arboretum or botanical garden.

✦ Create a website about a topic that is dear to you in regards to nature.

✦ Write a letter or email to your local politicians.

✦ Donate to a land or nature conservancy group or area you love.

✦ Write articles or letters to the editor in support of Earth.

All our relations

There is nothing more generous than a tree. A tree offers her hospitality to anyone who arrives: the black ant, the grey squirrel, the finch, raven, and red-tailed hawk. She sways in a deep dance with the air when he moves through her body, whether he is a breeze or his older brother, the wind. All these living beings mingle among her branches, which are literally and figuratively open to all new arrivals. During the cold winter she offers solid structure and a model of gestation and rest for us; in spring she offers her beauty and vibrancy. In the hot summer she offers shade and coolness, and in autumn she offers ripe fruit and can stun us with her red, orange, and yellow beauty before releasing it all to add richness to the soil.

What I have learned from the trees is to be conscious of what roots me well, and to cultivate these roots. I am sure you understand by now that the natural world nourishes me, and I spend as much time with her as possible. In nature, I learn to honour my inner rhythms by observing the passing of nature's cycles. There are times when my creative energy is vibrant, but more often as I age I notice times when I need to honour my body and simply rest. This responsiveness to what is calling lessens my stress and loosens anxiety's grip. My prayer is that you, too, can walk with Earth in reciprocity and love. And, that through this, you find your heart filled with colour, your mind and body at ease, and your imagination, intuition, and creative energy deeply informing you.

> **"Nature's peace will flow into you as sunshine flows into trees. The winds will blow their own freshness into you, and the storms their energy, while cares will drop off like autumn leaves."**
> — *John Muir, 1901* (Our National Parks)

References

Abram, David. (1996). *The spell of the sensuous: Perception and language in a more-than-human world*. New York: Pantheon Books.

Berry, Thomas. (1988). *The dream of the Earth*. San Francisco: Sierra Club Books.

Blake, William., & Baskin, L. (1968). Auguries of innocence. New York: Grossman Publishers.

Buzzell, Linda & Chalquist, Craig. (2009). *EcoTherapy: Healing with nature in mind*. Berkeley, Ca: Counterpoint.

Carson, Rachel. (1965). *The Sense of Wonder*. New York: Harper Collins.

Davis, John V. (1998). The transpersonal dimensions of ecopsychology: Nature, non-duality, and spiritual practice. *The Humanistic Psychologist, 25*(1-3), 60-100.

Davis, John V. (2011). Psychology, transpersonal, and nonduality. In *The international Journal of Transpersonal Psychology studies. 30*(1-2), 2011, pp. 137-147, 30(1-2)

Harding, Stephan. (1997). What is deep ecology? In *Resurgence journal* Vol. 185 pp. 14-17

Harding, Stephan. (2006). *Animate Earth: Science, Intuition and Gaia*. White River Junction, VT: Chelsea Green Publishing Company.

Ingerman, Sandra. (2000). *Medicine for the Earth: How to transform personal and environmental toxins*. New York: Three Rivers Press.

Louv, Richard. (2008). *Last child in the woods: Saving our children from nature-deficit disorder*. New York: Workman Publishing.

Macy, Joanna. (2003). *World as Lover, World as Self: Courage for global justice and ecological renewal*. Berkeley, CA. Parallax Press.

Macy, Joanna & Brown, Molly Young (1998). *Coming back to life: Practices to reconnect our lives, our world*. Gabriola Island, BC, Canada: New Society Publishers.

Morrison, A. L. (2009). Embodying Sentience. In Buzzell, L. & Chalquist, C., *Ecotherapy: Healing with nature in mind*. (pp. 104-110). San Francisco, CA: Sierra Club Books.

Muir, John. (1901). *Our National Parks*. New York: The Riverside Press.

Olsen, Andrea. (2002). Body and Earth: An experiential guide. Middlebury bicentennial series in environmental studies. Hanover, NH: Middlebury College Press.

Rilke, Rainer Maria. (1996). *Book of Hours: Love Poems to God*, Barrows, A. & Macy, J. (Translators). New York, Riverhead Books.

Roszak, T., Gomes, M., & Kanner, A. (Eds.) (1995). *Ecopsychology: Restoring the Earth, healing the mind*. San Francisco: Sierra Club Books.

Scofield, B. & Margulis, L. (2012). Psychological discontent: Self and science on our symbiotic planet. In Kahn, P. & Hasback, P. (Eds.), *Ecopsychology: Science, totems, and the technological species* (pp. 219-240). Cambridge, MA: The MIT Press.

Sewall, L. (2012). Beauty and the Brain. In Kahn, P. & Hasback, P. (Eds.), *Ecopsychology: science, totems, and the technological species* (pp. 265-284). Cambridge, MA: The MIT Press.

Sewell, Louise. (1999*). Sight and Sensibility*. New York: Tarcher/Putnam.

Resources

Video

Ribbons of Sand: www.youtube.com/watch?v=utDERYua404
A love letter to wilderness: http://www.karmatube.org/videos.php?id=6932
David Suzuki Foundation: One Nature: https://www.youtube.com/
    watch?v=ah0csZUtFHs
The Great Bell Chant: https://vimeo.com/6518109
Meet Barry Lopez: https://www.youtube.com/watch?v=hY6XMIGkohA
Earth Hour: https://www.youtube.com/watch?v=2UywrjnOaUE
Joanna Macy: The great turning: https://vimeo.com/ondemand/greatturning

Websites

Chopra Center (www.chopra.com/)
Daily Good (www.dailygood.org/)
Earth Empathy (http://www.earthregenerative.org/earth-empathy/resources.html)
Ecotherapy Heals (with newsletter) (www.ecotherapyheals.com)
Earth Hour (www.Earthhour.org/)
Gratefulness (http://gratefulness.org/)
On being with Krista Tippet (https://onbeing.org/)
The works that reconnects (https://workthatreconnects.org)

Books

Abram, David. (2010). Becoming animal: An Earthly cosmology. New York:
    Pantheon Books.
Berry, Thomas. (1988). *The dream of the Earth*. San Francisco: Sierra Club Books.
Berry, William. (2010). *Leavings: Poems*. Berkeley: Counterpoint.
Brady, M. (2009*). Right Listening*. Langley, WA: Paideia Press.
Hillman, James. (1992). *The thought of the heart and the soul of the world*. Putman,
    Conn. Spring.
Hillman, James. (1995). A psyche the size of Earth: A psychological foreword. In M.
    Gomez, A. Kanner & T. Roszak (Eds.), *Ecopsychology: Restoring the Earth, healing
    the mind* (pp. xi-xvi). San Francisco: Sierra Club Books.
Hutton, M. (2003). Listening to the land. In M. Brady (Ed.), *The wisdom of listening*
    (pp. 243-260). Somerville, MA: Wisdom Publications.
Loori, John Daido. (2005). *The Zen of creativity: Cultivating your artistic life*. New York:
    Ballantine Books.
Macy, Joanna. (2006). The Work that Reconnects [Training DVD]. Gabriola Island,
    B. C., Canada: New Society Publishers.
Macy, Joanna & Johnstone, Chris. (2012). *Active hope: How to face the mess we're in
    without going crazy*. Novato, CA: New World Library.
O'Donohue, J. (2004). *Divine beauty: The invisible embrace*. LOCATION: Random
    House.
Olsen, Andrea. (2002*). Body and Earth: An experiential guide*. Lebanon, NH:
    University Press.

Plotkin, Bill. (2003). *Soulcraft: Crossing into the mysteries of nature and psyche.* Novato, CA: Publisher Group West.

Roszak, Theodore. (1995). Where psyche meets Gaia. In M. Gomez, A. Kanner & T. Roszak (Eds.) *Ecopsychology: Restoring the Earth, healing the mind* (pp. xi-xvi). San Francisco: Sierra Club Books.

Swimme, Brian & Berry, Thomas. (1992). *The universe story: From the primordial flaring forth to the ecozoic era — a celebration of the unfolding of the cosmos.* San Francisco, Calif.: HarperSan Francisco.

Suzuki, David. (1997). *The sacred balance: Rediscovering our place in nature.* Vancouver, BC: Greystone Books.

Tredinnick, Mark. (2005). *The land's wild music: Encounters with Barry Lopez, Peter Matthiessen, Terry Tempest Williams, & James Galvin.* San Antonio, TX: Trinity University Press

Vaughn-Lee, Llewellyn. (Ed. 2013). *Spiritual Ecology: The cry of the Earth.* Point Reyes, CA: The Golden Sufi Center.

EcoPsychology educational resources

Sofia University Certificate in Transpersonal EcoPsychology. www.sofia.edu/academics/tec/

Naropa University Masters Degree in EcoPsychology. https://www.naropa.edu/academics/masters/ecopsychology/

Pacifica Graduate Institute Degree in Community Liberation and EcoPscyhology. https://www.pacifica.edu/degree-program/community-liberation-ecopsychology/

Institute for Earth Regenerative Studies. www.Earthregenerative.org

Lewis and Clark College EcoPsychology Certificate. https://graduate.lclark.edu/departments/counseling_psychology/ecopsychology/

Yoga and Anxiety

Angie Davis

I love Angie. She is my yoga teacher. I think she is an angel. On her web site profile I read about how yoga helped her heal. I had no idea to what depth she meant until I asked her if she would like to contribute to this volume. She enthusiastically said she could write a chapter and a story. Here is her chapter and following on page 218 is a riveting heartfelt story of her journey. Namaste.

— Elke

Yoga helps different people for different reasons. If you feel drawn to yoga, chances are high that it has something to offer you.

My own love of yoga is vast and deep. After going through a life-changing traumatic fall, many things are helping me to recover. I have shifted and changed through trying different techniques, therapists, and healing modalities, but yoga has always been there as the one stable guiding force of healing for me. It has always offered me something on my healing path.

I had already been practicing yoga for about five years before my fall, but when I got healthy enough, coming back to my mat was one of the things that saved me. I literally stepped out of hiding in closets onto my yoga mat. Just arriving to breathe and gently move, again and again and again, helped me calm my mind and nervous system. The breathing, the postures, and the safety of yoga helped me feel my body and my world again, very slowly and very safely.

In the broken and scattered pieces of my life after loss, yoga has been the glue that has allowed me to paste some of those pieces back together in the image that is becoming my new life. The comfort of practicing in community, but on my own mat, the repetition of movements and cueing of breath, body, and thoughts, the gentle instructors who hold space, and the subtle energy shifts after class all helped me feel a desperately needed sense of safety when my world was confusing and blurry. I have arrived at the studio in such a heightened state I could barely talk to anyone, I have cried for a solid hour through class, I have stayed in one position while the class has moved on just to try to be with emotions that come up... and through it all, I have kept coming back. Because yoga continues to teach me to slow down, feel my body, be aware of my thoughts, and take care of me. It helps me peel away the layers of physical, mental, and emotional tension brought about by my trauma and anxiety. It reminds me time and again: less gripping, more softening.

Why yoga?

We know that with anxiety the nervous system is on high alert and that this chronic stress response can leave us feeling physically depleted, mentally scattered, and emotionally overwhelmed. Meditative practices can calm an overactive brain. Since anxiety is a future-focused emotion, anything that keeps you in the moment is helpful. Practicing asana (physical yoga practice), pranayama (breathing practice), and mindfulness/meditation can relax and restore an anxious system.

When I speak in this section about yoga, I really am talking about yoga as a practice that includes all three of these aspects of physical practice, breathing practice, and meditation practice. It is impossible to separate out the three, which is why yoga is often referred to as a meditation in motion. We use the tools of yoga to train our brains to be present and be with all of our experiences, so that we experience them fully and move from one moment to the next with a sense of strength and present-moment focus.

As you enter into or continue a yoga practice, know that consistency matters. "Every day, a little, and often," is a guiding principle to go by. Start small and keep it manageable. Also know that you can practice yoga in various positions (lying down, sitting, standing), settings, and times of day. Yoga can also mean just getting yourself into one pose and staying there.

Try out different tools and techniques and see which ones work for you at different times and in different situations. A habitual yoga practice can help you stay calm in daily life, respond, rather than react, to life events with strength and feel deeply connected to yourself and the world around you.

Eight ways yoga helps us manage anxiety

As a practice that cultivates and strengthens our ability to be in the moment, for those of us with anxiety yoga can:

✦ Soothe our nervous systems.

✦ Help us understand and welcome the functions of the body, mind, emotions, and senses.

✦ Give us tools to respond to the events in our lives with less anxiety.

✦ Teach us about healthy living choices through yogic philosophy.

✦ Assist us in breaking cycles of repetitive negative thinking, self-criticism, doubt, anxiety, and worry.

✦ Improve the quality of our sleep.

✦ Anchor us to a deep groundedness and sense of well-being within ourselves.

✦ Support us in moving beyond just treating the symptoms of our anxiety and help us learn effective coping strategies for our own unique body and mind.

✦ Through all of these benefits, yoga can help you greatly improve the quality of your life.

How yoga centres us

1. Yoga opens us to self-compassion

Any self-care practice begins with curiosity and compassion. This is your practice, your time, your experience. The goal is for you to be curious about sensations, feelings, thoughts, emotions, and anything else that arises in your yoga practice. Having compassion for yourself means releasing judgments about your experience, such as letting go of feeling like other people are looking at you in a yoga pose, not worrying about how a certain pose "should" look and not being hard on yourself about having a mind that wanders in meditation (everyone's mind does!).

A yoga practice is about teaching yourself that you care about yourself, that you are willing to show up for you. There is no good or bad or right or wrong in any aspect of your practice (physical practice, breathing, meditation). You are not trying to fix or change your reality but are more working to accept it as it is, welcoming everything as a messenger that tells you if you are on or off course. Yoga teaches you to accept yourself whether you are on or off your mat, even as you strive for more depth in all areas of your life. It also trains you to be with discomfort, experiencing and witnessing it rather than running from it. Being with what makes you uncomfortable on your mat can help you face the things you are anxious about off the mat. Remember: curiosity and compassion! You will get to know yourself more and more, softly, with each breath!

2. Yoga teaches us to be the witness

Our minds wander. They are supposed to. The mind has a thought-producing function. In yoga, you learn to watch the mind wander without being caught in it. You watch in order to develop the witness. Developing the witness function of your mind strengthens your ability to bring your mind back to a point of focus (breath, mantra, body sensation, etc.). You learn to bring your mind back over and over again. Over time, you slowly learn to catch the wandering mind and bring it back more quickly. A common analogy in the yoga world is that you are the sky and your thoughts are the passing clouds. You learn to watch the clouds without judgment and attachment, in time witnessing them and letting them float on by. As you develop the ability to do so, you begin to get a strong sense of the vast, solid, unchanging part of you. In essence, you learn that while sensations and thoughts (the clouds) come and go, you are at your core the solid blue sky. Getting in touch with this unchanging part of yourself puts you at ease and helps you develop the confidence to face any life situation.

With anxiety, this watching and witnessing can feel difficult at the start. To help, you can anchor your focus with something tangible such as the feel of your breath in your body, counting quietly in your head, or the repetitive sound of saying a mantra. Essentially, you give the mind something to do to bring it to stillness.

3. Yoga trains us to have a present-centred focus

The worry that underlies anxiety is an emotion of the future. The practices of yoga and meditation can help you learn to be in the present moment, slowing down your spinning mind and the feedback loops of feeling overwhelmed and worried it likes to get into. Strengthening your ability to pay attention to how your breath feels in your body and how your body feels in poses keeps you firmly anchored in the present moment. Learning to be more and more present in poses over time develops your awareness. With this developing awareness, you bring on board both the witness function of your mind and a sense of inner peace, a deep knowing that no matter what your outer circumstances are, you have a deep well of grounded, unchanging well-being within you. Over time, this deep sense of groundedness and well-being becomes interwoven into every moment of your practice and daily life.

4. Yoga puts us in touch with our bodies

The physical practice of yoga (asana) increases body awareness. We begin to learn to experience physical sensation as a messenger. Think of sensations as supporters that are helping us respond to the sensory information that our bodies are constantly sending us. Our job is to sense, welcome, and respond to this information. In this way, as we grow in our ability to sense our bodies, we also develop our attention, concentration, and relaxation response, which lowers physical tension and stress both on and off the mat. We develop greater physical and mental relaxation, calm and soothe our central nervous systems, and grow the body's natural sense of resiliency. In addition, through regular asana practice, we improve our ability to feel and witness tension in body and mind, and thereby increase our ability to let that tension go, bringing about action through awareness.

A consistent physical practice can help us learn the subtle messages our bodies are sending us, the early signs of stress and anxiety, effectively preventing the body from having to shout at us through heightened anxiety, panic attacks, and/or going into other hyper-arousal or freeze responses in order to make us listen and respond to it. Additionally, with an anxious body and mind, our systems tend to constrict. Yoga helps us relax, be aware of, and lower, the physical tension, and soften the hold anxiety can have on us.

5. Yoga puts us in touch with our breath

Grow steady in your breath and you'll quickly discover peace of mind and freedom.
— *Yogavasishtha, 10th Century AD*

We take an average of 24,000 breaths a day, many more if we're active. Breath is closely linked to every function of the body and mind, including the digestive and circulatory functions, vital signs, muscle tone, mental and emotional states, and thoughts and feelings. Breathing patterns change to match our physical states and physical states change to match our breathing patterns. With stress and anxiety, most people resort to a pattern of upper chest breathing. This type of breath is short, shallow, and irregular, and makes us feel tired, fearful, and over-reactive, partly because of the over-production of cortisol that is associated with this type of breathing.

Conversely, whole body breathing that is deep and slow helps us feel relaxed and able to respond rather than react to our experiences. In particular, taking long, rhythmic exhalations reduces fear and anxiety and promotes the overall health of our system. Deep breathing produces serotonin and oxytocin, our feel-good hormones.

Through regular deep breathing and specific pranayama exercises in yoga class, we can develop breath awareness, expand lung capacity, and strengthen our breathing muscles, which all helps to clear the mind of the worrisome thoughts that anxiety feeds on. As we learn to focus on our breath through a variety of poses, so do we learn to focus on our breath through a variety of life experiences anywhere off of our mat. It is important to remember not to think about our breathing, but to really sense and feel the experience of breath in your body. Simply put, our breath is a powerful healing resource.

6. Yoga makes us aware of our thoughts

Thoughts have a powerful effect on the body and the body has a powerful effect on thoughts. A consistent yoga practice trains the mind to stay in the present moment. As we learn to do so, we begin to become more aware of our experiences in the present moment. As we become more aware, we can be the witness more often and, without judging, see the thoughts and patterns in our minds. We can strengthen our ability to witness our present experience, which can include seeing early thoughts of worry and anxiety. As we begin to see these early thoughts, we can prevent them from getting worse by taking actions that support health, either changing our thoughts or responding to them through movement. In this way, purposeful thought begins to replace worry. As we practice letting go of the worries by bringing our minds back to our bodies and breathing sensations, we can begin to be less attached to and create more space from our thoughts.

Thoughts are just things to be aware of. They are constantly changing. If we try to run from our thoughts, they often recur as they try to get our attention. Thoughts are messengers too. They are trying to give us information about steps we can take to be balanced and healthy. Through yoga, we can learn to slow down to listen and take positive actions that will help break our loops of negative thinking.

Just as physical sensations are the messages sent to us by our bodies, think of thoughts as the messengers sent to us by our minds. We have more than 12,000 thoughts a day, of varying quality and nature. By learning to welcome and understand both positive and negative thoughts as messengers, we can find new patterns of thinking that help us develop a friendly relationship to anxiety and to feel generally more positive and in control.

7. Yoga is a spiritual practice

Simply put, yoga means union of mind, body, and spirit. Even if you look at yoga as a completely physical practice, your mind and spirit are also being shaped by your physical asana practice. Every time. Whether you know it or not, these three components are always at work in a yoga class.

You are a spiritual being having a human experience. Yoga can become a way of life that helps bring this side of yourself to the surface. Through yoga, you can learn to be deeply connected to yourself and everything around you, to have faith that you have the resources to meet and greet any moment with the proper response, and to experience your underlying wholeness. The yoga path can help you heal your suffering, align your actions to be in harmony with your values and purpose, and open to your sankalpa (your heartfelt mission in this life). Yoga is a path of awakening and devotion to living your best, most soul-filled life possible. Will you get on your mat today?

Yoga tools to support you in studio and at home

Breath

When working with your breath, get to know yourself and what works and doesn't work for you. There is immense power in the breath to help calm your anxiety. Do know that sometimes taking big gasps of air can increase your anxiety. Slow and steady breathing is important. Try different techniques when you are calm and when you are anxious. As with anything, experiment and see what works best for you.

Following are three simple and easy breath-work strategies that can help you regulate the flow of air in your system, which in turn quiets racing thoughts, slows your heart rate, lowers your blood pressure, relaxes your muscles, and gets rid of toxins while allowing you to fill up with fresh oxygen. Overall, breath work creates balance and ease in your mind, body, and emotions.

The techniques are fast and effective, and all they take is a little practice. You don't need a yoga teacher or a yoga studio, and you can practice in your car, in the bathroom, quietly in a meeting, pretty much anywhere and any time you feel distracted or stressed and need to soothe your system.

1. Lengthen exhale. One of the simplest ways to work with your breath during times of anxiety is to concentrate specifically on lengthening the exhale. Make sure when you practice lengthening your exhale that you do not go beyond your own ability to exhale at length, which would cause you to gasp for air. Focus on developing a smooth transition from inhale to exhale and exhale to inhale, and if you feel the need to gasp at all, shorten your exhale.

Most people are naturally comfortable with a 6-count breath, a 3-count in for the inhale, and a 3-count out for the exhale. Begin with this count for a few moments, 3 in and 3 out. Begin to slowly deepen your exhales until you make your exhale twice as long as your inhale, gradually building up to a count of in for 2, out for 4. Practice for 30 seconds, then increase to a minute or two, then to several minutes. The counting in and of itself is calming for your mind as well.

2. Square breathing. The pattern of square breathing is inhale, hold, exhale, hold, repeat. Begin with a count of 3, counting quietly in your head: inhale 1, 2, 3, hold 1, 2, 3, exhale 1, 2, 3, hold 1, 2, 3, and repeat. As you become comfortable with the pattern, increase your count to 4, 5, 6 or beyond. Just keep the count the same for each round, so that your inhales, exhales, and holds have the same duration. Steadiness of breath equals steadiness of mind.

3. Alternate nostril breathing. "Nadi Shodhana," or alternate nostril breathing has a few variations, and each can be practiced in a seated position. It may seem confusing at first, but it's just a simple pattern based on the square breathing pattern, which you will master quickly. A hint that may help as you open and close your left and right nostrils is that you always exhale then inhale through the same nostril.

Leaving your left palm somewhere comfortable on your thigh or lap, raise your right hand. You need your thumb and ring finger for this. You can place your index finger and your middle finger between your eyebrows or curl them in and let them rest in the air.

Place your thumb over your right nostril, closing it. Breathe in through the left nostril for a count of 4, hold at the top for a count of 4, then remove your thumb. Close your left nostril with your ring finger, exhaling through your right nostril to a count of 4. Hold your breath for a count of 4. Inhale through the right nostril, pause for 4 at the top, release your ring finger, close your right nostril with your thumb, and exhale for 4. Repeat and feel free to change your count, but again always keeping it the same duration.

Hint: Remember to exhale and inhale through the same nostril and then switch fingers.

A quick YouTube search will give you visual supports with the second and third technique as you get to know them. Remember to practice often during both calm and anxious states.

Poses

Hundreds of different yoga poses offer hundreds of different benefits. Some are universal and some are unique to individuals. You have to find what feels best for your mind and body. In general, beneficial poses for those of us with anxiety are calming forward bends and grounding reclining poses. Repeating the same poses, and giving our bodies and minds time to arrive and settle in these poses, is also beneficial. So try doing the same poses over and over again, hold them for longer, and as you hold focus on your breath.

1. Forward bend sequence. Try these poses out on their own or as a little mini sequence.

Seated cross-legged forward fold

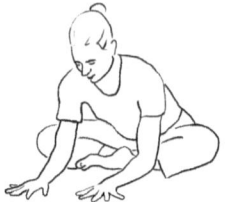

Cat/cow movements: hold cat at least twice as long as cow

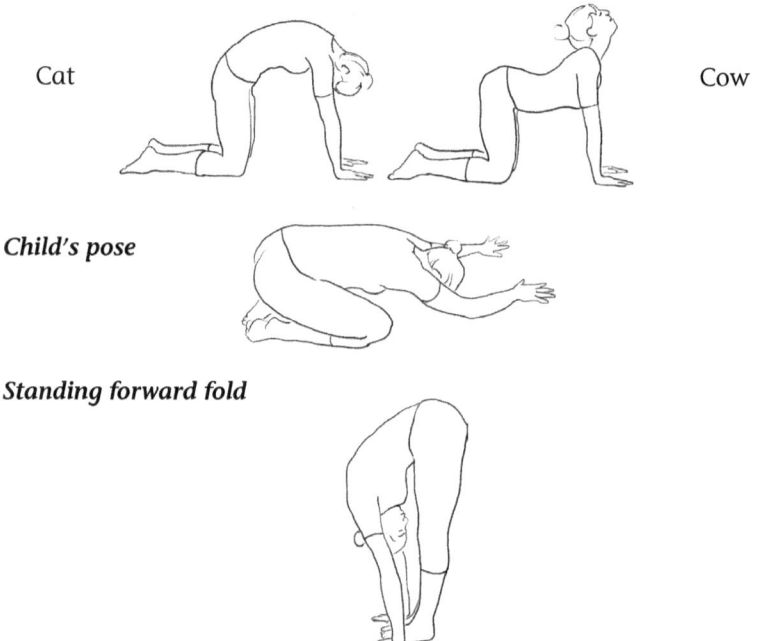

Cat   Cow

Child's pose

Standing forward fold

Choose from seated wide-legged forward fold or seated head-to-knee forward bend, on the right and then the left side

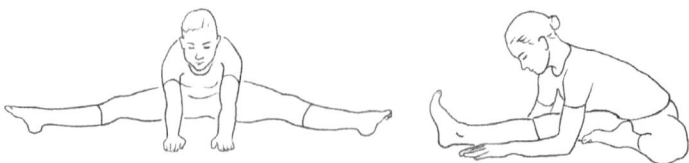

2. **Reclining sequence.** Reclining poses connect your body to your mat and to the Earth. They can feel very soothing, but you need to be careful about being too open and triggering your anxiety. Listen to your body and do what you need to do to feel comfort. If anxiety arises in savasana, for instance, change it by turning on your side in the fetal position or make yourself feel more protected by weighing yourself down with props. Props can feel very calming at any time, but especially when you feel unsettled, anxious, or stressed. A buckwheat bolster feels very grounding, but a large bag of rice can replace it for those starting out or on a budget. Place the prop on your chest or belly in reclining poses and note how your body and mind respond.

Happy baby pose

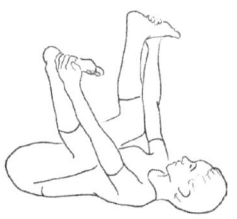

Reclining bound-angle pose (supta badha konasana)

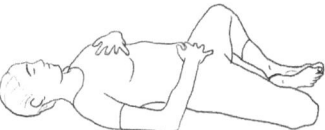

Reclining twist with knees stacked

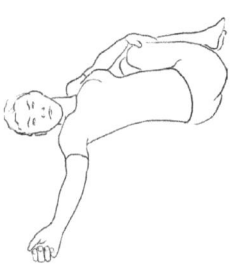

Legs up the wall pose (viparita karani)

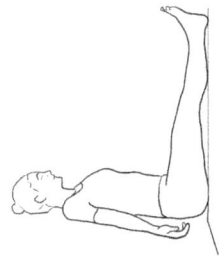

Corpse pose (savasana)

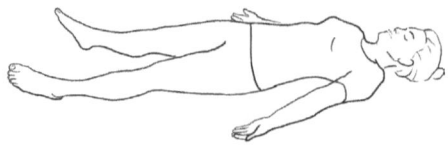

In addition to forward bends and reclining poses, here are five more poses that I find particularly calming. I practice these on their own for an extended length of time. Get into them, get so comfortable you don't need to move a muscle, and then give your body and mind at least 20 minutes to calm and settle.

3. Thirty-degree angle pose (also known as elevated chest pose) with burrito arms. This one takes a bit of work and some prop and blanket gathering, but it is my absolute favourite pose for calming my entire system. The images give you the best set-up for doing this at home. Here are a few extra pointers:

You always want your forehead to be higher than your chin, so prop up your neck and the back of your head with blankets.

Bring your tailbone right to the bolster before lying back. If your bottom is feeling bony and uncomfortable, give yourself extra padding by sitting on a blanket.

Getting into burrito arms will be the last thing you do when you set yourself up for a 30-degree angle pose. Place a blanket across your chest, wrap it around the backs of your upper arms, then take your right hand across to the left and tuck the blanket under your upper arm and elbow and do the same with the left arm on the right side. It should be snug and comforting. Think of a baby being swaddled. It is easier to do burrito arms on yourself with a heavier blanket, such as a Mexican blanket. You may also leave your hands by your side as shown below. You may also leave your hands by your side as shown below. If you don't have the props available for this pose yet, a nice alternative is the "legs over a chair" pose.

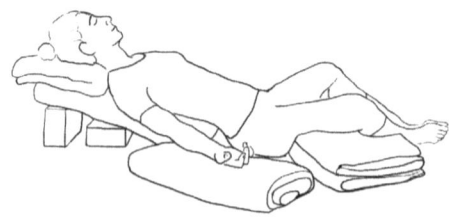

4. Crocodile pose.

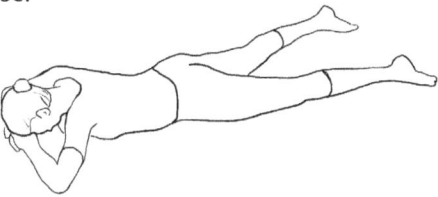

5. Savasana with bolster on top of chest.

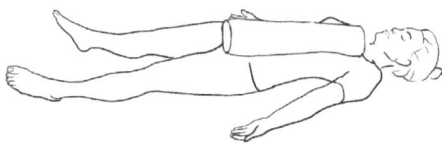

6. Legs up the wall pose.
Try a bolster or bag of rice on
your belly as you rest here.

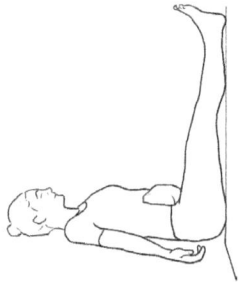

**7. Supported seated (in a chair or back against the wall) or lying
down butterfly hug.** For the butterfly hug, take your right arm across
your chest. Place your right fingertips into the side wall of your left
chest on top of your ribs and let your right hand rest on your chest,
keeping your fingertips pressing into your side ever so slightly. Take
your left arm across your chest and press your left fingertips into the
centre of your top shoulder line and let your left hand rest on your collar bone and upper chest.

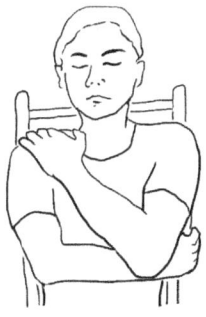

Meditation

Yoga is mediation and meditation is yoga. Through the practice of yoga you train your mind to return to the present moment over and over again. If you are searching for a meditation practice, one particular yogic practice that has helped me with trauma and anxiety is yoga nidra. Yoga nidra is compared to yogic sleep. It trains your mind and body to go into brain states that are similar to sleep, allowing you to deeply rest and restore yourself. Yoga nidra calms and rewires the subconscious mind, which can help soften and soothe anxious thoughts. There are also various branches of yoga nidra styles, which you can find on YouTube. Also try searching for my favourite style, *iRest yoga nidra*, by Richard Miller.

New to yoga?

Yoga is a 5,000-year-old practice. Since its inception, many lineages and branches have developed so that today there are hundreds of different types and styles of yoga. The practice of yoga involves learning about your body and mind, and what does and does not work for you. So instead of describing the types and styles of yoga or trying to convince you that one or another is better for you, let's talk about the ways in which anxieties can get in the way of going to a yoga studio, and how to get past them.

"I don't know what to do in a yoga studio!" Feeling a little lost as a person who is new to a yoga studio is to be expected. It's okay. Here are a few things that will help you understand what is happening.

Most yoga studios will have an entrance area, separate from the actual studio, where you can leave your outdoor gear and belongings (shoes, coats, purses, etc.) and register for class. Once you've done these things, enter the studio and set up your mat. Ask the instructor or another student how to set up your mat. Or, if this worries you, plan to enter a few minutes before class so you can simply follow what others do as they set up their mats. How people behave in the studio is different from studio to studio. Some studios have a strict no-talking policy, while in others people chat in low voices until the instructor comes in. Your best bet may be to set up your mat and lay down to start getting centred through your breath. Just notice it and feel it as you lie there and other people set up for class. Close your eyes if it feels safe for you and helps you focus on your own experience.

There are tools or "props" we use in yoga class to help us with certain poses. The most common props are a block, a strap, an eye bag, a blanket, and a bolster. You may be directed by the instructor on how to use a prop. They are also there for your physical and emotional comfort. During your practice, you can take whatever props you want at any time. Play and experiment. Remember always that what happens on your mat is for you: your comfort, your enjoyment, your mind, body, and spirit. Find the things that make you savour your time on your mat. If this means an eye pillow over your eyes in lying-down positions, a blanket under your bony knees in tabletop poses, or a block to lean on in balancing poses, then do it. It's okay.

It's okay to not resonate with an instructor. Every yoga instructor is different. Try many, find the ones you like. Some give instruction only on physical alignment, while others also give you mental, emotional, and/or spiritual things to think about and ponder in your practice. Personally, I crave instructors who speak to my soul during class. You absolutely must find instructors that you respond to. Otherwise, you will stop going.

On a yoga studio schedule, there are many different kinds of classes. There will be descriptions of these classes on the studio's website. The only way you are going to know what it's actually like is to try it out with different instructors. One instructor may have you moving very quickly and powerfully in a vinyasa class, while another may have a much slower pace.

Be comfortable with being uncomfortable. There will be new words and new ways to move your body. You will not understand some of it, and this is a completely common experience. Don't worry, after only a handful of classes you will understand most of what is happening. Part of the beauty of yoga is in its repetition.

If you are brand new to movement, know that beginning to tap into and feel your body may feel strange at first. You might not know how to have a relationship with this container that is with you every day. You may feel uncomfortable, giddy, or reluctant to do it. These are all just ways your body releases tension as you begin to strengthen your mind-body connection.

Emotional stuff will likely come up. Regardless of the instructor's style, yoga will always be working on your mind, body, thoughts, and spirit. During your practice, unresolved issues may arise. This, too, is normal. Yoga is loved by so many partly because it helps peel away these layers of stress and emotion that we carry.

Everything shifts and changes. In relation to yoga, this means that your body will feel different on different days. A pose will feel slightly different each time you do it. Your thoughts may be quiet, busy, scattered, or serene depending on the time of day and what is happening in your life, and your emotions may ebb and flow too. The practice of yoga gives you space and time to notice all these shifts and changes so that you can learn what they are and how they feel. Becoming more aware of these shifts and changes, the normal ebb and flow of everyday living, puts you more in touch with that part of yourself that does not change, the core of you that is solid and stable.

Know that if you're still feeling fear and anxiety about going to a yoga studio, there are other ways to build your confidence so you feel ready to come to a yoga studio. Start at home by following YouTube videos or on various yoga and fitness apps. You can also book a private session for yourself or a small group of friends, either at your home or in the studio. Private sessions will allow you to learn some of the cues and names of poses, while you also see how an instructor leads a class.

Anxiety during class

We've discussed the benefits of yoga, yoga poses that may help for anxiety, and issues and concerns of those who are new to yoga, so now let's talk about what happens if anxiety arises in yoga class. Whether you have mild anxiety or an anxiety disorder, you will likely experience anxiety on your yoga mat. It's okay, this happens to everyone. Here are some things you can do.

Remember that your number one priority in your yoga practice is to take care of you. First and always, you come first, not following what the instructor says word for word. If anxiety arises during your practice and you need to change what you're doing or stray from what the class is doing, then do it. Change the pose, slow down, speed up, or go into a pose you know is comforting. Honestly and truly, your yoga instructors want you to do this.

Know that as yoga teachers we want you to be in class, no matter what your mental, physical, or emotional state happens to be. A woman I met once told me about an absolutely beautiful yoga journey she had been on. Near the beginning of her recovery from a significant, entire-body physical injury, she found a yoga teacher who encouraged her to come to class even though she could not even do any of the poses yet. This woman lay in savasana (resting pose lying on your back) for the entire class. Her practice was visualizing and imagining in her head that her body was going through the motions during the class. This too is yoga. Gradually, over months and years, she was able to join in and do more and more of the movements. Whatever place you are starting from is perfect and wonderful and most definitely welcome in yoga class.

Keep in mind that in a yoga class, we do not all need to look the same. You may feel this has to be the case when you begin, but your instructors want you to learn to listen to your own body, which includes changing it up and doing what you need to do to care for your mind, body, and emotions. I honestly feeling like shouting, "Hallelujah" when a student skips or does something different from what I am saying in class. It means they are deeply listening to their mind, body, and spirit.

Don't leave your outside world outside when you come to yoga class. If you have things that help you with your anxiety—affirmations to read, a stone to hold, an essential oil to put on your forehead—bring them to practice with you and use them as needed. Whatever calms you off the mat can also calm you on the mat.

Remember your breath. Come back to your breath. Focus on your breath. Extend your exhale. Do square breathing.

Visualize in a way that helps you. You might visualize sending energy down through your feet, blasting energy out through your heart as light into the world, or any other visualization that helps you feel grounded and stable.

Use your time on your mat to loosen the ties of anxious and fearful thoughts by practicing being the witness. Observe your thoughts and emotions as waves of sensation rise and fall through your physical practice. Begin to witness instead of judging your thoughts and emotions. As you develop the ability to do so, you strengthen your ability to pause and take skillful action in response.

Conclusion

Namaste is often said at the end of a yoga class. In simple terms, it means the light in me sees and honours the light in you.

To you I say, Thank you for your presence, your reading of my words, your openness to learning about befriending your anxiety and the anxiety of others. My heart is full of gratitude that you are exploring the inner world of the mind and the possibilities yoga may offer for healing and health. Peace and Namaste.

Resources

"Integrative Restoration Institute" website by Richard Miller: https://www.irest.us/products/source#

Managing Anxiety and Stress with Kundalini Yoga

Susan Allen — Sat Akal Kaur*

It was at the Toronto Yoga Conference where I heard this beautiful soulful chanting and learned about Kundalini Yoga and that Muskoka has our own Kundalini instructor Susan Allen—Sat Akal Kaur. In the event that you get a chance to try this yoga, try a few sessions as each session is very different as there are hundreds of Kriyas. Sat Nam.

— *Elke*

Kundalini Yoga means uncoiling yourself to find your potential and your vitality and to reach for your virtues. There is nothing from outside. Try to understand that. All is in you. You are the storehouse of your totality.

—*Yogi Bhajan*

Why Kundalini Yoga is a part of my life

Kundalini yoga and meditation help us develop a relationship with our true selves. Being disconnected from our spirits opens us up to stress. When we are not connected, a gap forms. In this gap we become

---

* Sat Akal Kaur is my spiritual name, which I received in May 2014. "Sat" is truth. "Akal" means undying, infinite. "Kaur" is a name that all women receive—the Princess/Lioness of God who walks with grace and strength throughout her life. Yogi Bhajan taught that every woman has the potential to attain this divine state, and encouraged all to manifest it. Living the truth is never limited by time and space and has always existed, exists now and shall always be. That is Sat Akal Kaur. Experience it and live it. Be who you are... be the truth. In this divine state of consciousness, many will feel uplifted.

ungrounded, stressed, and unhappy. A relationship with the self gives us confidence and understanding. When we have this connection we can be happy, fulfilled, and stress and anxiety free.

Yogi Bhajan says, "Happiness is our birthright."

For me, nothing has given me this feeling of calmness like Kundalini yoga. The more I study, the more the picture comes together and becomes clear. The practice is so practical and fulfilling that I wonder why it took so long for me to find it. In my late 40s and early 50s, I suffered from depression and was constantly searching outside myself for relief. I embraced many things—Hatha yoga, Nia, mindfulness-based stress reduction, and all kinds of group programs for long periods of time. I had wonderful teachers but nothing gave me a feeling of contentment or belonging. I often felt that I was on the edge, but never quite getting there. The feeling that I was looking for came to me in my first Kundalini yoga class.

On a physical level, I have greater stamina and flexibility, and on a spiritual level the connection I now have with myself is much deeper and growing.

About Kundalini Yoga

Yogi Bhajan, Master of Kundalini Yoga and Doctor of the Psychology of Communication, brought the science of Kundalini yoga and meditation to the West in 1968. This was the first time in history that Kundalini yoga and meditation were taught to the public. This ancient technique, considered the yoga of awareness, had been practiced in secret in his homeland. It wasn't shared with common people, as the upper class believed it could give them power. Yogi Bhajan referred to it as the "householders yoga" and believed that the technique needed to be accessible to everyone. He often remarked that he was in the West to create teachers to share the gifts of the teachings, not to collect students.

The profound effects of this powerful practice can bring you in healthy ways to a higher state of knowing and awareness. Yogi Bhajan realized it was what we would need coming into the "Age of Aquarius." The new age of knowing, the shift from the Piscean to Aquarian Age, occurred in 2012. He saw people desperately looking to expand their consciousness through drugs, alcohol, and other unhealthy habits. It is said that Woodstock was opened with a Kundalini yoga practice, led by a person who had practiced in Los Angeles with Yogi Bhajan.

> Kundalini yoga means "awareness."
> Awareness is a finite relationship with
> infinity. That's all it means. This dormant
> energy is in you. This awareness is sleeping
> so you only experience (a limited part
> of) your full capacity. When it can be
> extended to Infinity, you remain you! In
> that state, nothing is lacking. This is the
> basic human structure, the framework
> through which we have to function.
>
> — *Yogi Bhajan*

Kundalini yoga is a science, and focuses on the experience the individual has during the practice. The direct experience you have with your breath, your body, and your life depends on what you are looking for. Kundalini yoga allows you to become the recipient of its gifts. They may be love, intuition, prosperity, awakening, physical practice... you take what you need.

Kundalini yoga and meditation have given me tools to strengthen my nervous, immune, and glandular systems. When the stress of today's lifestyle overtaxes a nervous system, it can lead to anxiety and depression. Through meditation and mantra I've raised my inner vibration to a higher level. From a spiritual perspective, vibration is considered to be the basic emanation from which all matter, energy, and consciousness are created. Raising our vibration brings us closer to merging with the highest vibration of all, the vibration of the universe.

Yogi Bhajan gives us the five sutras of the Aquarian Age

✦ Recognize that the other person is you.

✦ There is a way through every block.

✦ When the time is right, start, and the pressure will be off.

✦ Understand through compassion, or you will misunderstand the times.

✦ Vibrate the Cosmos. The Cosmos shall clear the path.

When we study and understand these words life become less of a challenge and more joyful. My personal favourite is the third sutra. When I become overwhelmed with work and life and don't know where to start, if I just start somewhere I immediately I feel relief. Doing nothing is much more stressful and causes additional anxiety.

Knowledge, happiness, purity and piety cannot be achieved from outside. They are always within you.
— *Yogi Bhajan*

This is true. Everything we need is inside us. It can be a long journey to realize this. I became part of a women's empowerment group. The group opened my eyes and gave me courage to discover I was not alone, that other women were struggling too.

We can develop our vitality. Get in tune with the five elements, the Tatvas: Water, Fire, Earth, Air, and Ether. Look at the beauty around us, feel the wind in our hair and on our faces, plant our feet firmly on the Earth, feel the deep emotional flow of life, connect with our internal fire. We become our own stress free zone. When we understand this we have the key to our own happiness and we live in gratitude. Kundalini yoga and meditation open us up to the possibilities of this awareness.

Kundalini yoga practices to alleviate stress and develop vitality

Tuning-in

Every Kundalini yoga practice begins by tuning in. This connects us to our inner teacher and the lineage of teachers who have gone before us. We carry on the golden chain of teachers and teachings. We chant the bij (seed) mantra: "Ong Namo Guru Dev Namo," which means: "I bow to my own inner teacher; I bow to the golden chain of teachers that have gone before." The vibration of the mantra and the meaning help connect us to our own inner teacher and to the universe of teachers that is part of the golden lineage of teachers.

Breath, pranayama

Pranayam, or pranayama, is the science of breathing consciously, controlling the movement of prana or life force through the use of specific techniques. Most people don't breathe properly; their breathing is shallow. Breath gives life; the deeper you breathe, the more fully you experience life.

> **The main problem in the world is stress. It is**
> **not going to decrease—it is going to increase. If**
> **through pranayam the shock can be harnessed,**
> **the entire stress and disease can be eliminated.**
> — *Yogi Bhajan*

Kriya

A kriya is a series of postures put together for a specific effect on the body, mind, or spirit. They can include physical postures and movement, breathing exercises, mantras, the sacred sound currents repeated aloud or in silence, and mudras, which are movements or poses.

There are thousands of kriyas. You may want to open your heart, strengthen the adrenals, warm up your spine, increase vitality, get rid of elementary fear, hidden anger, or subconscious patterns... there is a kriya for everything.

The kriyas below can be found online through the Kundalini Research Institute: http://kundaliniresearchinstitute.org, and 3HO, The Happy, Healthy, Holy Organization Yogi Bhajan founded in 1970 (www.3ho.org). The Yogi Bhajan Library of Teachings is constantly being added to.

Pittra Kriya

This kriya relieves stress, balances the chakras, and keeps the sympathetic and parasympathetic nervous systems balanced and strong.

Kriyas for relieving your elementary stress

+ Kriya for releasing the elements.

+ Kriya to take away stress.

Mantra

> **What is a mantra? Mantra is two words: "Man" and
> "tra." "Man" means mind. "Tra" means the heat
> of life. "Ra" means sun. So, mantra is a powerful
> combination of words, which, if recited, takes the
> vibratory effect of each of your molecules into the
> Infinity of the cosmos. That is called "Mantra."**
> *—Yogi Bhajan*

Mantras are a creative projection of the mind through the vibration of sound; the tongue stimulates the meridians of the mouth's upper pallet to release endorphins. When I do this, it increases my intuition, takes me out of my head, and brings me to a neutral space. I found that the more I practice, the more the mantras come into my head automatically. This is a great stress reliever.

Mudras

In the Kundalini practice, Mudras are hand positions that lock and guide the flow of energy and relax the brain. Each part of the hand relates to a certain part of the body or brain and affects different emotions or behaviours. Each of our fingers relates to a different planetary energy. When we stimulate these energies we get specific effects.

By curling, crossing, stretching, and touching the fingers and hands, we can talk to the body and mind as each area of the hand reflexes to a certain part of the mind or body.

Some commonly used mudras include the following. In each mudra, exert enough pressure to feel the flow of energy through the "nadis" (psychic channels) up the arms, but not enough to whiten fingertips.

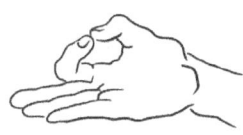

Guyan
The tip of the thumb touches the tip of the index finger, stimulating knowledge and ability. The index finger represents Jupiter, and touches the thumb, which represents the ego. Guyan Mudra opens us to calm.

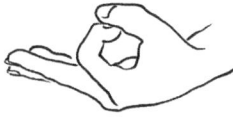

Active Guyan
Bend the index finger at the first joint, and tuck under the thumb, add pressure to the finger nail to activate knowledge and intuition.

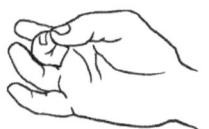

Shuni
Tip of middle finger (Saturn) touches the tip of the thumb, stimulating patience.

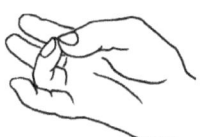

Surya or Ravi
Tip of the ring finger (Uranus or the Sun) touches the tip of the thumb, for health, energy, and intuition.

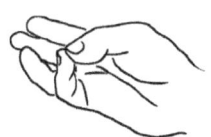

Buddhi
Tip of little finger (Mercury) touches tip of thumb for intuitive communication.

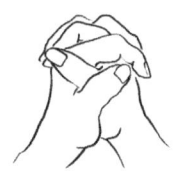

Venus Lock
Interlace fingers with the left little finger on the bottom, with the right thumb on top for men and the left thumb on top for women. The Venus mounds at the base of the thumbs are pressed together to create glandular balance, focus, and concentration.

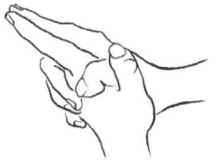

Jupiter
Point the two index fingers (Jupiter) together. This focuses energy and good luck and expands to break through barriers.

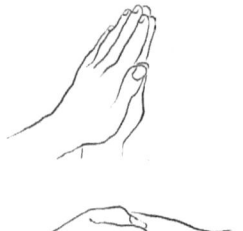

Prayer
Palms are pressed firmly together, stimulating glandular secretions. It's a grounding and meditative mudra.

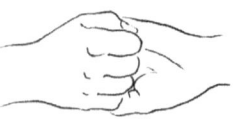

Bear Grip
Left palm faces out from the body with the thumb down. The right palm faces the body, with the thumb up. The fingers are curled and hooked together to stimulate the heart and intensify concentration.

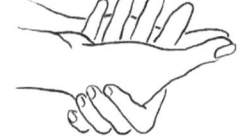

Buddha
Right hand rests on left for men, left hand on right for women, palms up, thumb tips touching each other in a gesture of reverence.

Relaxation

During a Kundalini yoga session, relaxation is as important to the practice as the kriya or meditation. Relaxation will bring you into a state of deeper meditation. It creates a time to integrate the mind and body changes that occur during the kriya.

Relaxation can be experienced by lying down and listening to mantra music or to a gong. The gong is an intervibratory system. It is the sound of creativity itself. Striking the gong creates deep relaxation and invokes thoughts and emotions. It stimulates the glandular system to higher functioning, opens the body, releases blocks, and stimulates circulation.

> The gong is the first and last instrument for
> the human mind, there is only one thing that
> can supersede and command the human mind,
> the sound of the Gong. It is the first sound
> in the universe, the sound that created this
> universe. It's the basic creative sound. To the
> mind, the sound of the gong is like a mother
> and father that gave it birth. The mind has no
> power to resist a gong that is well played.
>
> —*Yogi Bhajan*

Meditation

There are meditations for getting rid of fear, opening your heart, beaming and creating the future, alleviating stress, breaking your subconscious mask, developing courage, etc. Some meditations focus on breath, some have mudras, some have eye focus and mantras. Many combinations exist in the Yogi Bhajan Library of Teachings. Be sure to follow them exactly as written. It's best to practice with a certified teacher.

Meditation to strengthen the nervous system

This exercise is said to give the nervous system great strength.

Posture: Sit straight in a cross-legged position.

Mudra: Cup the hands slightly and clap them in front of the heart at the rate of one clap per second. Your hands must create a sound. Elbows are relaxed downward. Mudras are believed to affect the flow of energy in the body.

Eyes: Closed.

Breath: Breathe in rhythm with the motion of the hands through pursed lips, inhaling as the hands are spread, and exhaling as you clap the hands together. We can use our breath, which is our life force energy, to calm our minds and master our lives.

Time: Continue for 11 or 31 minutes. You choose the time. How long you meditate affects the outcome.

During the last two minutes, grip the hands together in front of the heart, tightening the hands as much as you can so that the energy begins penetrating your body. Breathe long and deep to control the energy.

To end: Inhale deeply, hold, and tighten your grip and your spine so that the energy goes through the entire nervous system. Exhale. Repeat two more times. Relax.

The success of the exercise depends on how much you tighten your hands during the last two minutes. If you feel dizzy following the exercise, drink some water immediately.

Closing a class

We close our practice by singing a blessing song. You can bless yourself, your family, your friends, your community, or anyone who needs it.

> May the Long Time Sun Shine Upon You,
> All Love Surround You,
> And the Pure Light Within You,
> Guide Your Way On

You can sing it three times if you wish. Then seal your practice by chanting "Sat Nam" three times. Sat is long and sounds like Saaaaaaat with a short Nam. Sat Nam means "I am truth, truth I am."

Simple practices to relieve anxiety and stress

Kundalini yoga and meditation as taught by Yogi Bhajan are excellent ways to gain strength, relieve stress, increase lung capacity, and uplift your spirit. Here are some simple practices you can begin with.

Cold showers

The easiest, cheapest, and most effective Kundalini yoga practice to boost our spirits is to take a cold shower. You may be thinking no way, but the benefits are many. Think about the feeling of jumping into a cold lake and how exciting, uplifting, and great you feel as your body adjusts and awakens to the experience.

Among the benefits, cold showers:

+ Increase immunity by speeding up metabolism, activating the immune system and increasing the white blood cell count.

+ Improve circulation. Capillaries open and the liver and kidneys flush toxins, and blood chemistry is balanced.

+ Stimulate glands, which promotes healthy secretions once the organs are flushed. Glands are the guardians of your health and youthfulness.

✦ Strengthen and reset the nervous system. When the parasympathetic and sympathetic nervous systems are balanced you feel energized and calm.

✦ Relieve anxiety and release endorphins.

Left nostril breathing

Simply close off the right nostril with the right thumb, and inhale and exhale deeply through the left nostril. This produces a calming effect, brings cooling moon energy to our system, and activates the right side of the brain.

Simple mantra: Sat Nam

"Sat" means truth and "Nam" means name or identity: truth is my identity. Simply repeating this mantra can ground us and connect us to the universal truth. Chanting this mantra increases intuition, balances the hemispheres of the brain, and creates clarity.

The original form of Sat Nam is Sa Ta Na Ma. These are the five primal sounds of the universe and the circle of life:

✦ Sa means infinity.

✦ Ta means life or birth.

✦ Na means death or transformation.

✦ Ma is rebirth.

✦ A is part of them all.

Yogi Bhajan says, "If you want to master something, teach it." Relating the teachings to others forces you to go deeper into all aspects of the practice. I love learning and have to admit that when I first was given my Aquarian Teacher Training Manual (the Level 1 Kundalini Yoga teacher training manual), I looked at it and thought, "This is the book of everything I ever wanted to know." What an exciting and fabulous challenge.

There are many dedicated teachers and practitioners working to preserve the teachings. If you are interested in finding a local teacher and class, the Internet is a great resource. There is a list of teachers on the KRI (Kundalini Yoga Research Institute) website. If you decide to join a class, it is recommended that you commit to at least six classes before you decide whether the practice resonates with you. Each class is different and so is the experience.

More resources on Kundalini yoga and meditation

www.yogibhajan.org/main/
www.spiritvoyage.com/sc/Kundalini-Yoga-Music/1.aspx
The Teachings of Yogi Bhajan. Published in Aquarian Times, Spring 2003.

The Radiant Fire:
Confronting the Critic and Nurturing the Inner Child

Krystal Demaine

I had the gift of being a participant in Krystal's workshop in the fall of 2017. There I found a way to comfort my inner child and make a promise to speak up and to look after it. Krystal's chapter gives us practical exercises that we can use to explore our inner child and critic. Bless her for sharing her work.

— *Elke*

Perhaps all the dragons in our lives are princesses who are only waiting to see us act, just once, with beauty and courage. Perhaps everything that frightens us is, in its deepest essence, something helpless that wants our love."
—Rainier Maria Rilke

Within the deep centre of every person lives an inner child. The inner child can be imagined as a physical representation of the self or as an imaginal felt sense. Sprightly into the world the inner child is born; pure, creative, and free. Freud referred to the inner child as the one who keeps an adult grounded and provides reminders of the true self.[1] Like an angel to the shoulder when in conflict, the inner child serves as the ever-present subconscious part of the self.

As an artist, mother, professor, and therapist, my thoughts are never far away from the role of the inner child. My own inner child can scream for attention in any aspect of my life. I often find the palm of my hand circling around my belly, physically soothing my inner child. I also crave gentle movement at the solar plexus, as if balancing a hula hoop, calming my own anxious feelings with a gentle swaying movement. The inner child, just like any child of the Earth, is bound for movement, play, release, and nurture. Just as we all do, the child can experience fear, anxiety, and the need for acceptance.

The inner child burns a fire that thrives in pure energy and freedom, but can also be smothered or silenced. Trauma, conflict, or ridicule of the child results in the cultivation of the inner critic. The critic, like the child, housed deep inside the core of self, can be easily provoked. Development of the critic may occur at any time in a lifespan, and can be engaged by a myriad of events. The critic can transform itself and strengthen its hold on the inner child, to impact self-image and the view of the world. The original critic may even extend its roots deeply to its ancestors, tapping into traumas not physically experienced by the individual. The unseen wounds of our ancestors who have experienced cultural or domestic conflict, neglect, or abuse may also fertilize the roots of the critic.

This chapter will explore the inner child, the critic, and their roots, and suggest exercises that I have used for myself as well as in professional practice, in order to nurture the child within. Nurturing the inner child can bring back a sense of wonderment, play, curiosity, and fulfillment that may have been lost or reduced by feelings of anxiety and stress. The activities are all presented in the context of play, imagination, and creativity as housed within and through the arts, and can be used for self-exploration, nurturance, growth, and discovery. It is important to process any difficult experiences that occur by way of engaging in this reading with the guidance of a licensed or certified creative arts therapist or licensed mental health clinician. Working with a therapist can engage clarity, understanding, and the tools to move through difficult situations. I encourage all readers to find creative solutions for living life to the best of their abilities and to draw upon meaningful resources for healthy living. I hope that you enjoy exploring this reading and find meaning in nurturing your inner child.

Authenticity

To feel is to be vulnerable.

—Brené Brown

Before we begin to explore roots of our inner self, our inner child, and our own personal narratives, we must start the voyage from a place of authenticity. This requires making a place for vulnerability. Brené Brown has suggested that all of life is vulnerable, that every human experiences vulnerabilities, and noted that, "Vulnerability is the core, the heart, the centre, of meaningful human experiences."[2] Robbins noted that when using the creative arts in healing "it is rare that our unconscious does not spill out," and that "accepting such vulnerability can offer a curative experience."[3] It has been long noted in nearly all spiritual beliefs that going inward, or looking toward the natural source, can allow for the deepest place of knowing. Art Therapist Pat Allen wrote an entire book on the use of art as a path for finding a way back to life. Her book, *Art Is a Way of Knowing*, has become essential to many arts-based healers and seekers, who are looking for creative outlets for exploring identity and art-making in everyday life.[4] Cultivating an authentic space and a willingness to be vulnerable is essential and to truly exploring the self.

Self-awareness

I have noticed that, in order to explore the self from an authentic place, there must first be a confrontation with the inner self and an acknowledgement of genuine thoughts and emotions. This means sitting quietly and listening to the self. This concept can at times seem hard to do, as our inner critic can get in the way of allowing ourselves to look inward. I give you permission to let go of self-judgment and allow yourself to sit and be.

One way of bringing this self-awareness to life is through mindfulness and meditation. In her writing on mindful meditation, Tara Brach[5] described a meditation group that was offered at a women's prison. One group member in particular, named Vanessa, was known as a bully among her peers. Vanessa protected some of her fellow inmates by intimidating and harassing others. In fact, Vanessa was a woman stricken by a history of torment and abuse, that without proper treatment had led to her legal sentence. One day, after the group heard a story by Buddhist Monk Thich Naht Hanh, Vanessa started to realize that she was not just the bad seed as she had always thought, but she was truly suffering. The acknowledgement of this suffering allowed her to be vulnerable, to be open, to explore, and to move toward personal change and ultimate acceptance. As a result, Vanessa stopped bullying. Brach's story shows the ability of mindfulness to bring awareness and personal insight to the ego. She has noted that all humans have the ability to tap into personal awareness. It is just a matter of finding the key to unlock one's vision. Insight can help drag a person out of their weakest moments and into a state of new health, integrated awareness, and compassion. Developing compassion must come with a state of personal awareness.

In addition to helping develop personal insight, mindfulness can also stimulate creativity. In this day and age of technological advances and busy schedules, there are many distractions that can sometimes overwhelm our ability to focus and attend to a single idea. According to Saitzyk (2013), mindfulness meditation can help to create mental space for new imaginative thinking, and thereby allow us to focus on what is personally most important. Meditation can also help create a starting point for new art, or enable us to view work from a fresh perspective[6]. Ultimately, meditation allows for us to become more attuned or aware of ourselves and our environment, which can be key to exploring our awareness of personal authenticity and vulnerability.

Equanimity

Authenticity and trueness of nature lends itself to equanimity, or equal balance from the inside out. In relation to vulnerability, Brown (2015), referred to a sense of trueness of self as an individual who is wholehearted, and described vulnerability as a component of being a wholehearted person.[7] In Eastern philosophy the balance of two polarities is essential to living life in harmony and fulfillment. The polarities can be represented as day and night, masculine and feminine, and warm and cold, or black and white, as in the yin yang symbol. Similarly, in Traditional Chinese medicine (TCM) there is an effort toward flow of chi—life force. Chi requires balance in five elements, sometimes related to colour, seasons, tones, organs of the body, and other worldly characteristics.[8]

In western psychotherapy and medical practices, people tend to seek help because there is a sense of feeling unbalanced or lacking in something. Looking at the whole self from an authentic place can help identify suffering and what's needed to work toward equanimity.

The inner critic

The inner critic, sometimes deemed the self-bully, like the one who jabs and throws punches at the internal character, can impact the lifespan. Therefore, discovering the origin of the inner critic deserves to be explored. Music therapist and psychoanalyst Louise Montello believed that it was important to confront the inner critic, examine the roots of its cultivation, and generate a dialogue to combat its bullying nature (Montello, 2002).

One client that I have worked with over the years discovered the fuel for his inner critic and was able to successfully confront the source. As a young boy, his brother, who was 11 years older, often teased him. When the older brother outgrew his toys, his brother received them often broken and tattered. Through exploring his inner critic, he recalled a memory from when he was six years old. His brother agreed to show him how his electric train set worked. The older brother set up the trains on the track and prepared the electric remote so that his younger brother could manipulate it. The boy waited in anticipation to have a chance, finally, to play with his big brother's toy—a toy that actually functioned. When he was given his turn, his brother triggered the remote with a quiet smile on his face, and all of the trains crashed and began to spark in flames. The big brother laughed and said, "Now look what you have done... you broke the trains!" Despite knowing that his brother had set up the trains to crash, the young boy convinced himself that he was to blame. This affected his self-esteem and his ability to stand up to superiors. His inner child was hurt, his critic was fueled, and the negative thinking impacted him into adulthood, which led to anxiety and eventually depression.

In her work on the area of performance wellness, Louise Montello[9] wrote that people have an innate ability to draw on essential musical intelligence (EMI), in order to "facilitate mind-body-spirit integration and radiant wholeness." (p.1). Montello asserted that such techniques as inner witnessing, dialoguing with the inner critic, and applying music relaxation/listening techniques can help enhance self-awareness and improve health. With undergraduate college students, Montello (2010) studied how stress-related issues, such as perfectionism, the inner critic, anxiety, stage fright, and self-esteem, affected the students. They attended Montello's performance wellness seminar, where they learned relaxation, breath work, meditation, and mindfulness techniques. Through these stress-relieving techniques the participants were able to transform what Montello referred to as polarized perfectionism and "disarm the inner critic."[10]

The emotional critic

The bullies of the world fuel the inner critic. As we age our skin gets thinner, literally and metaphorically, which allows physical and psychological poisons to seep more easily into our bodies. Quiet anger can wreak havoc on a soul.

Quantum physics describes how the environment plays a role on the inner workings of the human body. Since the human body is composed of approximately 70 percent water, and water absorbs energy, it is important to surround the body with healthy energetic feelings, people, places, and things. Japanese researcher and artist, Dr. Masaru Emoto[11] explained the role of emotions and our physiological response to it through his experiments with water and emotions. In his research Emoto exposed frozen petri dishes of water to various sounds, including music, spoken words, typed words, and videos. The crystallization that occurred through the freezing process produced different samples. Emoto found that when presented with what was deemed positive, the crystals formed complete and aesthetically pleasing shapes; alternatively, when negative sounds or images were presented, the crystals resulted in deficient and uneven shapes. For example, classical music produced whole crystal forms, while heavy metal music produced fragmented forms. Emoto's research concluded with the notion that sound and environment affect not only the human body, but the Earth as a whole. The Earth is composed of almost 70 percent water, which is necessary for the survival of human kind. With this knowledge, coupled with Emoto's research, it is important to consider the impact that kindness and compassion have on the human race and the planet we live on.

When the body is exposed to stressful or harmful situations, the firing of bodily chemicals (such as the stress hormone cortisol) doubles. Since 80 percent of the cortisol receptors are in the gut, we tend to feel anxious in our bellies. In our hearts, we can feel the rush of adrenaline increasing the natural heart rhythm, to a palpitation that can make it feel difficult to catch the breath. In the brain, neurologic structures can begin to change as the central nervous system compensates by rewiring with the fired chemicals. This internal and unseen altering can change the way we parent, work, live, and play. These unseen transformations are the neurologic and physiologic underpinnings of the inner critic. Knowledge of the internal works as a scientific basis for understanding anxiety, plays a significant role in the development of wellness programs, and in creative opportunities to cope with stress and anxiety.

The inner child

The inner child needs nurturing, acceptance, and understanding. The body and the self need to be educated in the emotions of the inner child by exploring the source of any pain or anxiety. The inner child needs to know that it is valued and worthy. Allowing for compassion towards the self and cultivating the inner critic are key to moving toward a whole and complete life.

Compassion specifically for the inner self is often overlooked. As we know, it is important to eat well, exercise, and drink plenty of water for good health. However, when it comes to nurturing the inner child, using childlike tendencies is key. Children are naturally inclined toward play, imagination, and creativity. Newborn children explore at a sensory level. When everything in the world is a new experience, food, the beach, air, the sun, animals, and nature all offer deep sensory exploration, creating the wiring of brain structures. Children initially explore sensory experiences slowly, innately mindful. As a mother of a young child, I remember when my son was learning to eat solid foods. I made him egg noodles. I remember him picking up a noodle, feeling its texture, looking, smelling, tasting, chewing the tiniest bite, and his eyes reacting by opening wide. Each step was slow and based on a sensory experience. We need to give our inner child permission to slow down, to do one thing at a time, and to notice each step of the way.

Our breathing has the ability to slow us down. A reminder to breathe, and to hear the words "I understand" when things feel stressful or overwhelming, is the best advice a person can receive. We have total control over the speed of breathing. While our hearts can sometimes seem to beat right out of our chests, breath has the power to slow down the heart's rhythm. Reminding the inner child to breathe, and to slow down, will offer the foundation for creative expansion, imagination, play, and centring.

Activities for the inner child and the critic

What follows is a series of activities that you can use to nurture and connect with your inner child. The child needs an opportunity to be heard and cared for, and allowing a place for creative expression will promote wholeness and wellness for your adult self. The activities begin slowly and deepen with the use of art materials and methods. Please give yourself permission to engage with these activities on a one-time or daily basis.

Heart listening

Begin this mindful activity by first finding a quiet place to sit still and close your eyes. You could sit upright in a chair or cross-legged on the floor with a cushion under your seat. Begin to breathe and find a natural breath. With your middle and index fingers joined together, locate your pulse in the wrist of your opposite hand, or in your carotid artery, to the right of your windpipe under your jaw. Listen quietly to your pulse and assimilate it internally. Breathe naturally and notice how the rhythm of your breath and the pulse of your heart intermingle. After a minute of listening quietly, bring your dominant hand to lie flat over your chest and heart area. Bring your non-dominant hand to the centre of your belly. Listen quietly to the pulses of your heart. Notice the movement of your belly. Allow yourself to breathe naturally and listen just. Stay here for as long as you like, allowing yourself to reconnect with your heart.

Visualizing the inner child

Prepare an unlined sketch pad and drawing materials. Sit quietly and begin to imagine what your inner body space looks like. Place your hand on your belly or your heart, and listen. Move your hand in a circle around your belly and notice any emerging sensations. Make mental notes of temperature, texture, movement, colours, sounds, dynamics, and any other expressions. Begin to draw the centre belly space on a sketch pad. Use the language of drawing to allow for freedom of expression. You may draw something abstract or concrete symbols, and accept whatever emerges. After you draw your inner belly space with all of its contents, describe in written language what you see, note the colours used, the location of those colours, the lines, shapes, forms, symbols, and anything else that is visually represented. Feel free to continue working on this activity for multiple days, or start over and create a new one. Accept whatever emerges on the sketch pad.

Music for the inner child

Make a playlist of music for your inner child. Begin with music that nurtured, inspired, and allowed you to feel safe; this music could span your entire life beginning from birth to the present. You can continue to add to your soundtrack over the course of your life. Allow yourself to feel free to move, play, cook, thrive, and live life with this music as your soundtrack. Share it with your children, and your children's children.

Collage for the inner child

Prepare materials for making a collage: magazines, scissors, glue, markers, an unlined sketch pad, and writing materials. Begin to identify images that you are drawn to and that are reminiscent of your inner landscape. What images animate your child? What landscapes allow you to feel free, playful, and at ease? Begin to draw and construct scenes where your child feels free and nurtured. Reflect on the images with a poem or other form of creative writing.

Inner child mirroring

With a partner, stand across from each other. Choose one person to be the leader and the other to follow. The leader will begin moving and the follower will mimic the movements. If you are the leader, imagine yourself existing in a smaller body, as a child. Notice how your body moves as you watch your partner copying you. Pause; notice how this feels. Then move from "child" back into the adult space of the body. Discuss with your partner how it felt as your body moved. Repeat the activity, this time as the follower.

Collage for the critic

Prepare collage materials: magazines, scissors, glue, markers, an unlined sketch pad, writing materials. Create an image of what the critic looks like. Perhaps the image is a collection of images, perhaps it manifests with a single image. Finally, create a picture of the critic or critics who helped to smother your inner child's fire. You may also add words and notes as to what the image represents to you.

Letter to the critic

After identifying the source of the inner critic through collage and writing, take some time to write a letter to the critic. Write everything that you would like to say, but can't say in person. Do not send the letter to anyone. Simply write it and save it in a private place. Writing the words will give you an opportunity to truly express how you feel in a safe, non-judgmental manner.

Mantra for the child

After looking at the body of work you have created through drawing, making a collage, listening, and moving, create or choose a symbol or gesture that represents your inner child. The gesture could be a short movement, and the symbol could be a sketch or painting. Give the symbol or gesture a mantra or positive affirmation. The affirmation could be something that starts with "I am..." Keep this symbol and mantra with you as a reminder of self-nurturance everything you have done to help your inner child. You may want to make multiple copies of your mantra to pin up in your home, or keep it in a safe private place that you can access when you need to reflect.

Conclusion

The inner child is the history keeper of human emotions, thoughts, and way of being—the child cultivated by the forces of nature, parents, siblings, and ancestors. While we may not have much control over the cultivation of the critic and the trauma to the inner child, we can reawaken the playful nature that allows the child to be free from pain, stress, and anxiety. Children are naturally inclined toward play and imagination. If we offer opportunities for creative play, we can, in turn, allow our inner child to radiate with joy and wholeness.

Each day we can create space to listen to and dialogue with the inner child. The arts can give us that opportunity of imaginative silent dialogue though reflective writing, creative meditation, drawing, and listening to the music that sparks the inner child's radiant light. To this world we arrive as children, peaceful and full of wonder and creativity, as well as a keeper of ancestral memory. Through playful art making we can rekindle our inner child, bring light to the roots of our pain and suffering, and move forward to a place of wholeness, joy, and peace.

Notes

1   Allen, P. (1995). *Art as a Way of Knowing*. Boston, MA: Shambhala.

2   Brown, B. (2015). *Daring greatly: How the courage to be vulnerable transforms the way we live, love, parent, and lead*. New York: Avery.

3   Brach, T. (2016). *True refuge: Finding peace and freedom in your own awakened heart*. New York, NY: Penguin Random House, LLC.

4   Demaine, K. (2015). Musical roots for healing: The five tone system in traditional Chinese medicine. In S. L. Brooke (Ed.), *Therapists Creating a Cultural Tapestry: Using the Creative Therapies Across Cultures (pp. 154-169)*. Springfield, Il: Charles C. Thomas

5   Emoto, M. (2011). *The hidden messages in water*. New York: Atria Books.

6   Freud, S. (2010). *Civilization and its discontents (complete psychological works of Sigmund Freud)*. New York, NY: W.W. Norton and Company.

7   Montello, L. (2010). The performance wellness seminar: An integrative music therapy approach to preventing performance-related disorders in college-age musicians. *Music and Medicine, 2*(2), 109-116.

8   Montello, L. (2002). *Essential musical intelligence: Using music as your path to healing, creativity, and radiant wholeness*. Wheaton, IL: Quest Books Theosophical Publishing House.

9   Rilke, R. M. (1984). Letters to a Young Poet. Trs. S. Mitchell. New York: Random House

10 Robbins, A. (1994). *A multimodal approach to creative art therapy*. London, UK: Jessica Kingsley Publishers.

11 Saitzyk, S. (2013). *Place your thoughts here: Meditation for the creative mind*. Los Angeles, CA: First Thoughts Press.

Resources

Freud, S. (2010). *Civilization and its discontents (complete psychological works of Sigmund Freud)*. New York, NY: W.W. Norton and Company.

Brown, B. (2015). *Daring greatly: How the courage to be vulnerable transforms the way we live, love, parent, and lead*. New York: Avery, p. 12

Robbins, A. (1994). *A multimodal approach to creative art therapy*. London, UK: Jessica Kingsley Publishers, p. 145.

Allen, P. (1995). *Art as a Way of Knowing*. Boston, MA: Shambhala.

Brach, T. (2016). *True refuge: Finding peace and freedom in your own awakened heart*. New York, NY: Penguin Random House, LLC.

Saitzyk, S. (2013). *Place your thoughts here: Meditation for the creative mind*. Los Angeles, CA: First Thoughts Press.

Brown, B. (2015). *Daring greatly: How the courage to be vulnerable transforms the way we live, love, parent, and lead*. New York: Avery.

I wrote this chapter on the relationship of traditional Chinese medicine healing and music therapy. Demaine, K. (2015). "Musical roots for healing: The five tone system in traditional Chinese medicine." In S. L. Brooke (Ed.), *Therapists Creating a Cultural Tapestry: Using the Creative Therapies Across Cultures (pp. 154-169)*. Springfield, Il: Charles C. Thomas.

Montello, L. (2002). *Essential musical intelligence: Using music as your path to healing,*

creativity, and radiant wholeness. Wheaton, IL: Quest Books Theosophical
Publishing House.

Montello, L. (2010). The performance wellness seminar: An integrative music
therapy approach to preventing performance-related disorders in college-age
musicians. *Music and Medicine, 2*(2), pp. 109-116.

Emoto, M. (2011). *The hidden messages in water.* New York: Atria Books.

Managing Anxiety
with Breathing

Dr. Colette Harman

I first met Colette in Kincardine 30 years ago. Recently she wrote a few books on managing anxiety and teaches a six-week program. This chapter is an approach that I am fascinated with and ready to try! I am delighted that our paths are travelling together again.
— *Elke*

In over 25 years of naturopathic practice, one of the techniques that really revolutionized my practice was understanding how modifying our breathing can help to effectively cope with and reduce anxiety. This came from training I received on the Buteyko Breathing Technique. The technique is named after a Russian doctor, Konstantin Buteyko. His interest in breathing began as a medical student in Moscow in the 1940s, when he observed that patients who were ill or in pain breathed more heavily than healthy people.

In his third year of medical school, Buteyko spent hundreds of hours monitoring patients' breathing as they approached death. As well, he asked other patients to hyperventilate, and observed a wide variety of symptoms, including anxiety, panic, asthma-like symptoms, high blood pressure, headaches, and even fainting. Interestingly, this same phenomenon was noted by a physician during the American Civil War, Jacob Mendez Da Costa. Soldiers presented with chest pain, heart palpitations, difficulty breathing, anxiety, and a variety of other symptoms. Upon examination, he found nothing physically wrong with these soldiers. These symptoms were referred to as "Soldier's Heart" and "Da Costa's Syndrome"—what we would probably call today Post Traumatic Stress Disorder (PTSD).

Through years of study and experimentation from the 1950s to the 1970s, Buteyko discovered that practicing "reduced" breathing reversed hyperventilation and eliminated related symptoms, including anxiety. He showed that how we breathe can either improve or damage our health, and that up to 90 percent of the population breathes more than is required for the activity they are performing. Why is this important? When you over-breathe or hyperventilate, you risk depleting your body's carbon dioxide (CO_2) pressure.

How carbon dioxide pressure affects us

Adequate carbon dioxide pressure in the bloodstream is essential for the proper functioning of the respiratory centre in the brain. Concentrations of carbon dioxide in our bodies are close to 20 times greater than in the air we breathe. If CO_2 pressure is high, the respiration rate (how many times you breathe in a minute) increases as a way of releasing excess CO_2; if the CO_2 pressure drops, the respiration rate decreases. This is how it is supposed to be if it weren't for the fact that most people over breathe all the time.

Why do we over-breathe or hyperventilate? When exposed to stress, the body elicits the fight, flight, or freeze response, in which adrenaline coursing through the body increases the breathing rate. However, once the stress passes, the body relaxes and resumes a normal breathing rate. Unfortunately, life in the 21st century is filled with lots of little stresses, with the occasional huge stress thrown in. This leaves the body with little opportunity to calm down and relax. Consequently, the respiratory centre in the brain responds by adjusting to this higher breathing rate as normal. Most people with anxiety can point to a specific stressful event or events as the initial trigger(s) causing the hyperventilation.

There is a cascade response in the body from this higher breathing rate and the resultant decrease in CO_2 pressure, which leads to poor and reduced oxygenation. Basically, when gas exchange happens in the lungs, the hemoglobin in the red blood cells binds to oxygen atoms and carries them to the rest of the body, where they are released to various tissues and organs. However, the red blood cells can release the oxygen only if there is enough carbon dioxide pressure to pull the oxygen away from the red blood cells. High CO_2 pressure causes an increase in the release of oxygen from the red blood cells to other cells of the body. Conversely, when hyperventilating or breathing more frequently than is required decreases CO_2 pressure, less oxygen is released to the cells of the body. These increases and decreases are known as the Bohr effect.

Low CO_2 pressure, known as hypocapnia, causes smooth muscle spasms, reduces oxygenation of the brain, and agitates the nervous system. What are the effects of these smooth muscle spasms? Smooth muscle wraps around all the hollow tubes of the body such as the airways, the digestive tract, the arteries, and the bladder. When the airways spasm, asthma results in some, and sleep apnea in others. When the digestive tract spasms, it can cause generalized bloating, flatulence, acid reflux, and indigestion. In serious cases, it causes the spasming associated with irritable bowel disease and in severe cases inflammatory bowel diseases such as ulcerative colitis and Crohn's Disease. When the arteries go into spasm it can increase blood pressure. If the coronary arteries spasm you have angina, and, finally, when the bladder goes into spasm it can cause urinary irritability and frequency, especially at night.

Among the effects of over-breathing or hyperventilation are anxiety and panic attacks due to lack of oxygen reaching the brain. Here are the most common symptoms of a hyperventilation attack:

✦ A "lack of air" sensation.

✦ Chest tightness or pain.

✦ Palpitations, pounding heart, or fast heart rate.

✦ Feeling dizzy, lightheaded or faint.

✦ Feeling "spaced out" or "not with it."

✦ Fear of dying, losing control or going crazy.

✦ Hot all over, sweating of the palms or armpits.

✦ Mouth feeling tight and forming an "O" shape.

✦ Tense muscles.

✦ Trembling and shaking.

✦ Visual disturbances, such as blurred or tunnel vision, flashes or shadows before the eyes.

✦ Nausea or stomach upsets.

✦ Numbness or tingling sensations in fingers or lips.

✦ Numbness and tingling of the face.

Many people think anxiety causes hyperventilation. The reality is that hyperventilation causes panic attacks, and chronic hyperventilation causes anxiety. The great thing is, you can change your breathing and stop hyperventilating, which stops the anxiety and panic attacks. The Buteyko Breathing Technique, when taught by a qualified Buteyko practitioner, instructs participants on how to retrain their breathing by doing breathing exercises on a daily basis.

To give you a sense of the benefits of the Buteyko Breathing Technique, I've provided three techniques which, when used as needed, can help you resolve panic attacks and even generalized anxiety. But first, more on preventing hyperventilation and anxiety attacks.

How to know if you are hyperventilating

Do you recognize any of the following six indicators?

✦ Breathing rate: Time your breathing rate by counting how often you exhale in one minute. If you exhale 13 or more times while at rest, you are hyperventilating.

✦ Deep breathing: Perhaps you breathe fewer than 13 times per minute, but if you are taking big deep breaths, you are hyperventilating.

✦ If you frequently yawn, sigh, cough, sneeze, or even hold you breath for seconds at a time, resulting in an irregular breathing pattern, you are hyperventilating.

✦ If you frequently mouth breathe, then you are hyperventilating.

✦ If you snore or have sleep apnea, then you are hyperventilating.

✦ If you have anxiety, then you are hyperventilating.

How you can reduce hyperventilation

Always try to breathe through your nose, not through your mouth, even with exertion and exercise. In a Buteyko class participants are taught how to exercise without mouth breathing. It takes practice but can be done. The nose is especially meant for breathing because the nose warms up cold air, cools down hot air, moistens dry air, and dries moist air. Furthermore, the mucous lining of the nose contains white blood cells that can zap any inhaled germs so that when the air reaches the lungs it is sterile and at body temperature. When you mouth breath, you bypass all that protection. We have a saying in Buteyko that you should breathe through your mouth as often as you eat through your nose. Definitely not recommended.

Many people who are mouth breathers have chronically stuffed-up noses, hence the mouth breathing. The less you nose breathe the more stuffed up the nose becomes. In essence, if you don't use it, you lose it.

There is a simple technique to unblock the nose, known as the nose clearing exercise:

✦ Sit up straight.

✦ After a normal exhale, close your mouth (if it's open), and softly pinch the nostrils closed.

✦ Gently and slowly nod your head up and down until you need to take a breath (usually six to eight times).

✦ Keeping the mouth shut, unplug your nose and inhale gently through your nose.

✦ If the nasal passages have opened slightly, continue to breathe gently through the nose.

✦ If there is still some nasal stuffiness, repeat the nose-clearing exercise as often as needed to maintain clear nasal passages.

Sometimes sucking a peppermint or inhaling the scent of essential oils such as rosemary, eucalyptus, camphor, menthol, etc., can assist in opening up the nasal passages. If this still hasn't cleared your nose, you may need to see a doctor to determine if there are any physical blockages such as nasal polyps in the nostrils or a deviated septum.

How to stop an anxiety attack

The following three techniques can aid in reducing and even halting hyperventilation, thereby reducing and even halting the anxiety. Each of these techniques involves holding your breath several times to break the cycle of hyperventilation. What makes them unique is that the breath holding is always done on the exhale, not the inhale as we are often used to doing.

1. The steps technique

This is done while walking, as when we feel anxious or panicky, we often want to move anyway:

+ Inhale and exhale normally several times while keeping your mouth closed (if possible).

+ On the next exhale, hold your breath for a count of 3 steps.

+ Resume normal inhaling and exhaling several times as you walk.

+ On the next exhale, hold your breath for a count of 4 steps.

+ Resume normal inhaling and exhaling several times as you walk.

+ On the next exhale, hold your breath for 5 steps.

+ Resume normal inhaling and exhaling several times as you walk.

+ Continue this pattern of breath holding and walking, each time increasing the breath holding by an extra step until you are holding your breath for a total of 10 steps.

At this point you may be feeling a bit calmer, in which case you could either sit down and focus on slowing your breathing to an 8 to 12 breaths per minute range, or do the following:

✦ Resume normal inhaling and exhaling several times as you walk.

✦ On the next exhale, hold your breath for 9 steps.

✦ Resume normal inhaling and exhaling several times as you walk.

✦ On the next exhale, hold your breath for 8 steps.

✦ Resume normal inhaling and exhaling several times as you walk.

Continue this pattern of breath holding and walking, each time decreasing the breath holding by an extra step until you are holding your breath for a total of 3 steps. If you are not completely calm by this point, repeat this whole pattern of breath holding and step counting 2 more times.

2. The counting technique

If you cannot or do not want to move or walk, then do the following:

✦ Inhale and exhale several times normally, hold your breath on the next exhale, and count to 3 (you can count as quickly or as slowly as you need).

✦ Resume normal inhaling and exhaling several times.

✦ On the next exhale, hold your breath for 4 counts (again as quickly or as slowly as you need).

✦ Resume normal inhaling and exhaling several times.

✦ On the next exhale, hold your breath for 5 counts (again as quickly or as slowly as you need).

✦ Resume normal inhaling and exhaling several times.

✦ On the next exhale, hold your breath for 6 counts (again as quickly or as slowly as you can).

✦   Resume normal inhaling and exhaling several times.

✦   Continue this pattern each time holding your breath
     for 1 extra count until you are holding your breath for
     10 counts.

✦   If you are feeling calmer you can then slow your
     breathing rate to 8 to 12 breaths per minute. If you
     aren't calm enough, then continue the pattern of
     breathing interspersed with breath holding on the
     exhale and reduce the breathing by 1 count, holding
     for 9 counts, then 8, then 7 until back down to 3 counts.
     If needed, repeat this pattern of breathing and breath
     holding pattern for another 2 times or until feeling calm.

3. The mini pause

This is a simple technique that can break the cycle of hyperventilation
and anxiety. The technique can be repeated dozens of times throughout the day.

✦   Inhale and exhale, and hold your breath for 2 to 5
     seconds. This should be easy and comfortable to do. If
     it's uncomfortable, hold your breath for a shorter period.

✦   Breathe normally, inhaling and exhaling several times.

✦   Inhale and exhale, and hold your breath for 2 to 5
     seconds.

✦   Repeat as often as needed until you feel calmer and have
     slowed your breathing to 8 to 12 breaths per minutes.

As well, the mini pause is an important technique to use whenever
you have a hyperventilation outburst such as coughing, sneezing,
yawning, sighing, and even laughing. Do a few mini pauses to replen-
ish the lost CO_2.

Practicing each of these techniques on a regular basis, especially
during times when you are not experiencing anxiety, will help them
become ingrained in your muscle memory.

Remember, anxiety is a symptom of chronic hyperventilation. You can reduce your tendency to hyperventilate, and the resultant anxiety, by mindfully nose breathing all the time. If needed, perform the nose clearing exercises as often as necessary to encourage nose breathing. As well, when at rest purposefully slow your breathing rate down to 8 to 12 times per minute. Finally, when experiencing anxiety know that you are hyperventilating and use any three of the anti-hyperventilation techniques described above in order to return to calm. There is nothing worse than feeling powerless and hopeless when it comes to anxiety. My goal is to give you these few easy and simple tools to give you back hope and control, so that eventually you can say goodbye to anxiety for good.

Guided Imagery:
How Your Mind Can Help You Reduce Pain and Cope Better with Stress

Dr. Roxanne Daleo

Roxanne, a.k.a. "Dr. Rosie," has been sharing guided imagery for many years. It is my pleasure to include her in this volume. Thank you for all that you do!

— *Elke*

A powerful form of mind-body medicine is now helping people of any age, including young people, to cope with both medical treatments and the everyday stress of life. Known as guided imagery, this effective method combines relaxation exercises, positive mental images, meditative breathing, and music to help us shift our focus from experiencing pain to coping with pain.

This is something I learned while working in a clinic research unit of a children's hospital in Boston, where patients from around the world came looking for hope. The risks were high and the treatments were horribly difficult. I witnessed firsthand the dramatic impact our minds and hearts could have on our health regardless of the prognosis.

Jake and Lucy's story

I could see the two small children through the window of the laminar air flow rooms as I made my morning rounds. This was the sterile environment in which I would conduct all play therapy and creative arts sessions for the duration of their bone marrow transplantations.

My daily responsibility was to allay the fears and anxieties of terminally ill children and their families. Also, I had to psychologically prepare them for upcoming medical and surgical procedures. I took the emotional rollercoaster ride along with them every minute of every day. For some children this involved at least three to four months in isolation; for others, up to two years. It wasn't easy. I could see them, they could see me, but I wasn't allowed to touch them in that sterile room.

The arrangement was two patients at a time, facing each other, separated by glass and clear plastic partitions. They waved to each other as the days went by. Even the young children had a deep knowing that they shared a common bond.

In the bed to the right of the flow room was a five-year-old boy by the name of Jake. In the bed to the left was Lucy, a nine-year-old girl.

Based on blood counts and the children's genetic make-up, the research team suggested that one child had an excellent prognosis for cure, while the other had a grave prognosis for survival. Yet, what ultimately happened had more to do with influences of attitude, mood and "live messages" they received and believed.

Jake's family was tight knit; his parents were present and Dad was a stable figure. His mom was an eternal optimist, and his older brother was the best matched donor for the bone marrow. They expressed deep spiritual beliefs. I often heard the mom say, "Jake, when you get out of the hospital we are all going to take you on a family trip to Disneyland!" This was the vision, the held belief, the "dangling carrot" Jake and his family kept hold of, which I dare say had energy of its own.

Lucy's mother visited every day, sometimes alone, sometimes with Lucy's older brother, a high school student. In Lucy's case, I never saw a father figure, and her mother appeared anxious and depressed most of the time, even though the doctors gave Lucy better reports for recovery than Jake.

I saw Lucy's emotional stamina decline more and more. I knew this from years of working with gravely ill children. They would lose their "spirit for play" and become emotionally closed. This was a warning sign that alerted me to Lucy's severe sense of hopelessness within her young soul.

Jack's mom sent him "live" messages every moment of the day. Lucy's mom gave her "depression" messages every day. I realized that I, too, was giving messages. With all my heart I gave each child "I am happiness, love, and the power of play," all wrapped in the invitation I

extended through creative self-expression, and an emotional inocula-
tion of compassion, and being present with passion and feeling.

You can well imagine the outcome for the two children. It was Jake
who had the poor prognosis, yet he lived and Lucy died. They confirmed to me that held beliefs about health, healing, genetic predispo-
sition to disease, even life expectancy are passed from one generation
to another. Further, the subtle energy of vibration of words and music,
resonating from the heart with clear intention, could have tangible
results.

Relaxation of the mind, body, and spirit is essential for everyone.
In today's increasingly complex and sometimes harried world, we are
more vulnerable to stress than ever. In fact, both positive and negative
events put stress on the mind-body system. Feelings of anger, worry,
nervousness, depression, and loneliness can escalate in anyone not
skilled in managing stressful events. Disconnection from our emotions
may be exhibited in physical symptoms such as headaches, changes
in eating and sleeping, and lowered immune responses, causing frequent infections.

Suppose you are faced with a situation that is unpredictable or out
of your control; for example, having an accident, feeling nauseated
from chemotherapy, or trying to sleep the night before your math
finals. Guided imagery will give you tools to put in your "medicine
bag" and pull out whenever you need them. They can help you relax
your body to a level where it can recharge itself. When you relax your
body, you decrease muscle tension and the stress that contributes to
physical and emotional discomfort.

You can use your mind to take an imaginary journey, far away from
the difficult situation (such as being in the hospital). Your imagination
is very powerful. Guided imagery offers a way to give your mind something positive to focus on through music, suggestions, and a guided
narration or story.

When you visualize, you transport yourself to a pleasant place as
soon as your eyes are closed. Unless you give your mind something like
this to focus on, it will decide what it wants to focus on and may choose
something like the pain. So practice directing the movies of your mind.
Tell yourself what you want to stay focused on, and your mind will listen and follow your instructions. Otherwise, you will have a mind with
a mind of its own. Where do you fit in? You must choose wisely to help
yourself get out of stress mode.

Creating a guided imagery setting

How do you learn guided imagery? You can be taught by a health professional or you can listen to audio programs created for this purpose. This is something I've created for my own clients. To make guided imagery work for you, here are important guidelines and ways to create the optimal atmosphere for relaxation.

✦ Choose a quiet space to elicit relaxation, such as an environment free of distractions like computers or mobile phones. Select a place that you can come back to again and again that is peaceful to you.

✦ Get into a comfortable position, sitting or lying down. You may want to use pillows or cushions.

✦ Just listen. Push "play": you will be guided through a series of exercises of relaxation. Just follow the storyteller. The narration is designed to have you become aware of your body and mind by engaging your imagination. Close your eyes, if you like. Breathe in and out naturally to soothe yourself. Keep your focus on your breathing.

✦ Establish regular practice. Consistency is the key. Choose one theme at a time and play it daily for several weeks, such as just before bed each night. Avoid listening to the playback immediately after eating, because relaxation lowers your metabolic rate and can slow your digestion.

✦ Use your imagination. Explore the process of combining listening with performing expressive arts activities such as drawing, painting, and writing. Remember, creativity is at its peak after listening and relaxing.

Here are four techniques that I've used to help my young clients apply guided imagery in creative ways.

Technique 1: The energy ball

+ Rub your hands together as fast as you can, while counting slowly to 30.

+ Put one of your hands up to your face, one centimetre (about ¼ inch) away. Feel the heat radiating from your hands.

+ Rub your hands together again.

+ If you can reach the painful body part, place your hand or both hands directly on it, or one centimetre (about ¼ inch) above it.

Imagine the warmth of your hand melting the tightness and pain, like the sun melting the snow on a rock. Breathe slowly and deeply, and send the breath into your hand. Feel how the warmth eases the pain.

Technique 2: Change your view

Pain is in the body and it is the mind that tells us about the pain—whether we're feeling a physical pain that is sharp or dull, or whether we're in a situation we think is hard, uncomfortable, or boring. It is possible for you to use guided imagery to learn to gain control of your feelings, thoughts, and judgments. You see, your brain makes no distinction between real or imagined information. Just take yourself to a scary movie and see how your body responds to the images on the screen. You may even feel your hands sweat and your heart race.

It is possible to turn off the inner chatter and reduce physical pain. You do this by learning to control your thoughts, feelings, and judgments about the pain. For example, you have probably said at times, "I hate this pain! I wish it would stop." This is an understandable response. (Try it right now and see.)

Is there another, more comfortable way? Yes. You can take some control by making a decision to let go of wanting things to be different from how they are right now. Stop fighting the pain or situation. Change your view: close your eyes and visualize an ocean. See the crashing waves reach the waterline. You can't stop the waves but you can learn to surf!

In any difficult situation you can tell yourself, "I can't take it any more," or "I can do this." Either way, your brain will follow your directions, so why not learn to master your mind so it can serve you in times of need? All it takes is determination. Say to yourself: "In this moment, there is something good I can focus on." This positive energy will automatically help your body, mind, and spirit.

You might ask, "How?" or "What's the point?" Well, how about focusing on the people who love you, rather than focusing on the negative things in life?

Focus on the expansive and open sky, stretching in all directions, blue, bright, beautiful. Imagine opening up possibilities. Now, imagine hooking your painful, unwanted thoughts to a white cloud and see them drift away until you can no longer see or feel them.

Technique 3: Expressive art symbolic gestures

+ Take out paper and paints or coloured pencils.

+ Draw a sky with white clouds on a 5cm x 5cm (2" x 2") piece of paper.

+ On the white cloud, draw a picture of your worry thought; or draw a symbol to describe your negative thought.

+ Take that cloud picture and crumple it up and throw it in the wastebasket.

By doing this powerful symbolic gesture, you are literally getting rid of your negative thoughts—getting them out of your head and throwing them away.

Technique 4:
From a grain of sand, I can make a pearl.

This is a multi-sensory expressive arts activity using an audio CD. You can download a sample of *From a Grain of Sand* at: http://drroxannedaleo.com/roxie/free-gift-request/

Materials

Paper (printed papers or construction paper) scissors, crayons, and an audio device for playing *From A Grain of Sand* music while designing your oyster shell and pearl.

How to make your shell

- ✦ Fold and crease an oval shape in half horizontally along the midline.

- ✦ Release and reopen the paper, then pinch together the small ends of the oyster seashell paper shape with the thumb and pointer finger of each hand. Simultaneously, push them inwards to meet each other vertically so that the fingers of your left and right hands meet each other as if you are tapping them together.

- ✦ Open and close them in this manner a few times.

- ✦ Release your fingers and the shape should hold itself together like a shell.

How to make your pearl

- ✦ Take a long, skinny strip of paper (coloured, white, pearl, or whatever you choose). Along the strip you can write or draw an "irritation"; something that is "bugging you." Beginning at one short end, roll it up into a ball, pushing the edges of the paper inward as you roll it so you can no longer see what you've written or drawn on the strip.

- ✦ Scrunch it tightly together in your hand and sing to yourself, *"Pearling is fun to do/I can turn it and grind it and smooth it... round and round and round it goes... until a pearl is formed,"* as you press it with your fingers. When you release it, the shape will stay together in a small ball, shaped like a pearl.

- ✦ Place your pearl inside your shell to remind you, always, that you are safe and well.

Remember, you are always using your imagination, and when you intentionally guide yourself to hold in your mind images of hope, love, and happiness, you will feel hopeful loving and happy.

In summary, if you use guided imagery you will see benefits of many kinds.

You will probably find that you are calmer, more relaxed, and sleep better. When you are being affected by something you can't control (like chronic pain or sadness), guided imagery can help you restore control and reduce feelings of fear, anger, impatience, and powerlessness. You will learn to see opportunities for replacing your negative feelings and thoughts with statements that are positive, strengthening, and hopeful. Guided imagery can help you change your focus and change how you manage stress. Use your imagination to guide yourself to health and happiness.

Open a child's mind to the Power Within. Find out more at: www.mindworksforchildren.com and www.drroxannedaleo.com

Boundaries

Elke Scholz

**You have a need and a right to love,
respect, and stand up for yourself.**

I am inspired to write about boundaries by what I witness in my personal and professional life: allowing boundaries to be crossed causes much stress, confusion, anger, and anxiety.

A healthy relationship with yourself and others has healthy boundaries. Healthy boundaries are a form of self-care and self-compassion. When it feels like others don't respect you, it is likely a clue to establish better boundaries or create some. Perhaps you need to respect yourself? All relationships have some kind of boundaries. Inner knowing of oneself is the first step to healthy boundaries. The following contains some guidelines for healthy boundaries.

Are you restless? Anxious? Agitated? Resentful? These are all signals to say that something is amiss. Perhaps you don't have healthy boundaries. Perhaps you do know yourself and your limits, however; someone is crossing them. Are you stressed in a relationship? Are you fed up with your neighbours? Or tired of office politics?

Healthy boundaries are important to a healthy and happy life. Setting and maintaining boundaries is a skill that can be learned, though sometimes we struggle with how to express our discomfort, to stand up for ourselves, and respect ourselves enough. What does all this actually mean? What does it look like when we are living it?

It could be the case when one person or situation crosses our boundaries or it could be a general way we allow actions to overcome us. Perhaps we are service workers (nurses, police, volunteers, caregivers, doctors, teachers, therapists, administrators, managers and so on...) and go past our energy limits, work through lunches and breaks; work overtime, do tasks we are not trained for or supported in, believing we are doing the right thing.

Another scenario: people around us ask many favours and we say "yes" even when we are tired. However, we do it out of obligation or a belief. Perhaps in a relationship the other wants to go further; although you are not ready, you give in and do it. Perhaps you are experiencing peer pressure to party or take substances you don't want to, and do it to belong or avoid confrontation.

> **Healthy boundaries means knowing and understanding what your limits are and expressing them and maintaining them.**

What are your limits?

Know your ethics, morals, and integrity. Know where you stand on issues. If you are unsure, perhaps reading and researching matters or talking with a friend will help with perspectives. Consider all aspects of your life, physically, emotionally, mentally, sexually, and spiritually. What can you accept, what makes you feel uncomfortable or stressed? Listen to your body.

Trust your body

Using the same 0 to 10 scale mentioned earlier on page 8 (zero being comfortable and calm, and 10 an almost unbearable feeling), consider your discomfort levels. Use the Yes/No/Maybe exercise. "YES" is obvious and "NO" is obvious. When does the in-between become uncomfortable? What number equals discomfort for you? (Reference Anxiety Warrior first book, page 137) Resentful? Painful? Too much? Sometimes we don't know exactly what causes the discomfort. And we don't necessarily need to know. No matter what, we can trust our bodily sensations. Sometimes we need to act right away. In introspection, we can assess.

Ask yourself: What is it about this interaction, or the other person's expectation, that bothers me?

As the discomfort continues, resentment festers inside us. Resentment festers when we feel violated or disrespected. We might continue to allow others to behave in a way that is not honourable or respectful. When someone's actions make us uncomfortable, it is a cue that they might be violating us or crossing a boundary.

Boundaries are personal. It does not matter that someone else may not be upset in a similar situation. What matters are your own limits and your limits need not be defended.

Trust your emotions

Anger, rage, hurt, disappointment, frustration, confusion, restlessness, withdrawal, guilt, and exhaustion are some clues that you may need to set a boundary. Complaining may be a habit we get into as a result of living past our boundaries. Feeling threatened, victimized, and suppressed can also offer valuable clues about boundaries you may need to set.

Practice self-awareness

When you are aware of what your limits are, that is when you can look after them. Understanding yourself, your feelings and your body, is the first step to honouring yourself. Your body knows when you have gone past your limits, or someone else has. See that as a signal, not as a weakness or flaw.

Consider your upbringing and past

How you were raised and your role in your family can become additional obstacles in setting and preserving boundaries. If you held the role of caretaker or people pleaser, you likely learned to focus on others and got used to ignoring your own needs, which would be draining emotionally, mentally, and physically.

It might please you to please others; however, is there a balance of self-care and self-compassion along with the serving? A life of service is a virtuous life, however not at anyone's expense.

In your relationships, is there a healthy balance?

Consider your work environment. What are the perceived expectations? No breaks or lunch breaks? Are there unrealistic expectations of workload and/or extra hours?

A high bar and standard are okay, however, with support and a team effort.

Give yourself permission

Fear, guilt, and self-doubt could stop us from speaking up. We might fear the other person's response if we set and enforce our boundaries. Saying no to an authority figure, a boss, a friend or a family member can feel intimidating.

Many believe they should be able to cope with a situation, or diminish their own discomfort and say yes because they want people to be happy with them and approve of them. Perhaps you compare yourself to others and their performance and endurance. Self-doubt creeps in and we question whether we deserve to speak up and have boundaries in the first place.

Boundaries are a sign of a healthy relationship and self-respect. Give yourself permission to set boundaries and put effort into preserving them.

Make self-care a priority

I remember when a dear friend said I had become boring and lacked my usual outgoing spirit. She said that I needed to take better care of myself. She was right; I was exhausted and lethargic.

I learned about self-care. If I was run down, how could I possibly do my best, give my best and be a quality friend, partner, mother, or business owner providing top-quality service? I learned that self-care is a priority so I can give 100 percent. When I have more energy and focus, I can give more. Self-care means so many things: healthy choices in lifestyle, living, sleeping, exercise, and eating habits. It includes listening to your body, your sensations, little niggles, intuition, and discomfort. All this is important in our well-being. There is a sense of calm and relief in our bodies with healthy boundaries.

Be clear, specific

You don't have to be nice to people who aren't nice to you. Use the NVC Model (pages 41–48) to understand your feelings and needs and to begin a compassion discussion. If this fails then continue in setting healthy boundaries. You cannot simultaneously set a limit with someone and also take care of their feelings: they may feel hurt, angry, or disappointed, but this is not your problem. Communicate as best as you can. Frame the boundary. Introduce your intent briefly. Be clear, and use specific limits and requests. Follow through with results and be firm.

Here are some examples: If you don't pick up your clothes they won't get washed. If you don't pay your share of the rent by (this date), then you will be moving out. Do your chores first and then I will give you a ride to town. If you want to eat here, bring groceries.

Maintaining healthy boundaries doesn't always require a direct and clear-cut dialogue. Some people get it or understand right away. With others, such as those who have a different personality or cultural background, you may need to be clearer and more direct about your boundaries. You may need to say and establish boundaries in several different ways. You may need to coach, explain, and teach people so they understand. In a respectful way, let the other person know what in particular is bothersome to you and how you can work together to address it. Give clear examples and be patient.

You will set boundaries when you are ready. Your body will let you know when things have gone too far or when you have given in too much.

Be assertive

Being assertive means standing up for your rights and for the rights of others. Not being assertive means allowing others to take away your rights. It's not reasonable to expect people to guess your limits or boundaries. Don't expect people to understand or comply.

Nobody can demand to know your mind or your business: what you share with others about matters that concern you is determined by what feels right to you, and not by what they want.

Nobody has the right to tell you what to think, though I have heard people say that they know what another is thinking. There is no conversation or communication in that.

No one has the right to tell you how you are feeling or should feel. You have a right to your own feelings, values, and beliefs. As humans we have a full spectrum of feelings. They just are, and do not need to be defended.

You have a right to be who you are and to live your own life harmlessly, regardless of whether others like it or not. You have a right to make choices and to have your own friends.

You don't have to feel guilty for not behaving as others might want you to, or for not giving others what they expect of you.

You have a right to your imperfections and shortcomings. You don't have to feel guilty for not being perfect. You are completely acceptable just as you are right at this moment, with whatever sensations, thoughts, and feelings you are experiencing.

You have a right to ask for what you need and to ask for help.

Creating a boundary is important. More importantly, we need to follow through for our well-being. You are allowed to say, for

example, "Don't use loud voices; I won't have it," or "I need you to
_____ because I need respect." If others behave poorly or trigger you, you have the right to tell them so, to ask them to stop, and to avoid them in the future if they choose to continue.

Seek support

If you're having a hard time with boundaries, seek support, whether that's a support group, church, counsellor, coach, or good friends. With friends and family, you can make it a priority with each other to practice setting boundaries together, to hold each other accountable, and to check in with each other.

Take small steps

Like any new skill, assertively communicating your boundaries takes practice. Start with a small boundary that isn't threatening to you, and then set more challenging and important boundaries.

**Setting boundaries takes courage, practice,
and support. It's a skill you can master.**

Transitional Poetry

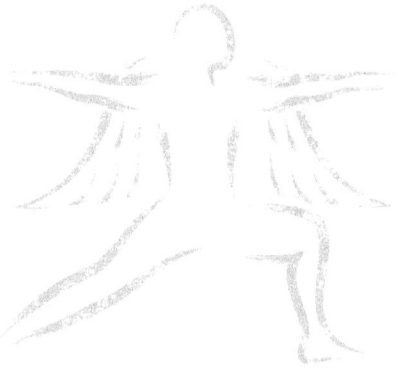

Transitional Poetry

The following are a few poems giving an expressive arts component to the book. I have written poetry since I could write words, and I sang songs before I could l write them.

The poems are a segue into the stories. The first poem is about what it sometimes feels like for me when I have anxiety. It is written in a slam poetry style. I have performed it several times. The second poem, by Reilly Scott, is her experience of seeking help. The third poem is a journey to health and groundedness. The fourth poem, by my daughter Emma Scholz Bertrand was posted on Facebook as I was putting this section together. Her passion and hope inspired me, as I hope it does you. It represents a shift in claiming her life her way. The fifth poem is an invitation to the reader.

The peace and quiet of DEAD
Elke Scholz

Retching guts, it sucks
I feel like a blender
Pin cushion, that'd be a treat
I feel like spikes in raw meat
To end or pause or rest from thought
racing — pacing — dicing — slicing —
This way, that way
— any way as long as I am asleep
The energy hurts until it stops
DEAD
DEAD

Dreams — nightmares — streams — scares
Uncover, blubber, tough
regretting every word,
insanely absurd inferred
To end or pause or rest from thought
racing — pacing — dicing — slicing —
This way, that way
— any way as long as I am asleep
The energy hurts until it stops
DEAD
DEAD

My blood is frothing
My sweat is fermenting
Lost dizzy fractured hoping
Vacant black thought, just coping
To end or pause or rest from thought
racing — pacing — dicing — slicing —
This way, that way
— any way as long as I am asleep
The energy hurts until it stops
DEAD
DEAD

A maze with no end
Reactions, actions
grinding my tongue — run away,
contradiction nails my lungs
To end or pause or rest from thought
racing — pacing — dicing — slicing —
This way, that way
— any way as long as I am asleep
DEAD
DEAD

Throat empty again
Can't breathe, I breathe too much
Ever tasteless, thorn I clutch,
ever wishing I can't touch
To end or pause or rest from thought
racing — pacing — dicing — slicing —
This way, that way
— any way as long as I am asleep
The energy hurts until it stops

DEAD

The inspiration for "Take this pill" came from my experiences trying to navigate the medical system with anxiety. Reflected in the poem are the feelings of deep shame and isolation that I have felt, culminating from years of direct and indirect messages received from a poorly equipped system that offers a very singular and biased perspective on treatment with no explanation or guidance towards healing. It was my hope, through the poem, that those who have had similar experiences might feel less alone in their battle and that we might begin to truly understand just how many of us go through this and how truly not alone we actually are.

Take this pill

Reilly Scott

Take this pill.
Don't ask why.
It doesn't matter.
I don't have time for questions.

Take this pill.
You are an inconvenience.
You've been here too often.
I don't have answers.

Take this pill.
I'll give you a blank stare.
I've never seen this before.
Words elude me.
I can't solve this.

Take this pill.
Why wouldn't you?
It's supposed to make it all go away.
I've been told.
A chemical imbalance, nothing more.

Take this pill.
What?
Serotonin. Genes are the cause.
Medication for life.

Now please stop talking,
you're making me think.

Take this pill.
Don't ask questions.
I can't believe you would try.
A deeper reason?
I've never heard of it.
It will shut your body up, I promise.

Take this pill.
It is the answer.
To think differently is crazy.
Why question the status quo?

Take this pill.
It's the only way.
It's all I can offer.
I've been trained.
Other ways of thinking are absurd.
Please step aside.
I am uncomfortable.

Take this pill.
You're taking too much of my time.
Can I make you go away?
There are so many of you.

I will never tell you,

so you will never know.

What is courage?

Elke Scholz

What is courage?
Is it facing a fear?
Is it making a decision,
just like that?

Or is courage...
a heavy knapsack
with stones picked up,
and turning stones over?

Or is courage...
letting the stream flow
gracefully over time?
Touching the earth?

Or is courage...
climbing that mountain,
flying in the wind,
slipping on a glacier?

Or is courage...
baring your soul,
daring to be seen,
letting others in?

Or is courage...
walking on coals,
feeling raw pain,
not giving in to rum?

Or is courage
believing in love?
Loving oneself?
Feeling another?

Or is courage…
having a child?
playing the child?
Having faith?

Or is courage…
standing strong,
singing our voice true,
accepting a gift?

Or is courage…
remembering again,
preparing to dig further
and allowing to live?

I'm in the second semester of my second year at university. For most of my life, I wanted to be a vet. I saved my money, worked every summer as soon as I could to save for seven years plus of university. However, after taking certain courses at university and working at a vet clinic I realized that being a vet was not in line with my values. My passions more wholistic and encompasses not only saving animals but also people and the environment. Then I became aware that being a vet would not make me happy. It would not make me feel like I was fulfilled with my life. This awareness began my journey of discovering my dreams and also kind of rediscovering myself. And on this journey, I wrote this on Facebook and my Mom asked if I would share it with you, so here it is.

Life Waiting for You

Emma Scholz Bertrand

Let go and you will be reborn!
Let go of the expectations of others
Let go of your own expectations about who you "should" be
Let go of your comfort zone, because we all know you aren't comfortable

Let go of the fear of changing your mind
Let go of the dreams that no longer resonate with you
Let go of the people who don't serve your higher self
Let go of your emotions, they don't need to stay
Let go of it all

Take in all the good energy that's around you
Take in people who lift you up
Take in the joy of doing what you truly love
Take in all that you need,

It's out there waiting for you

Soul Destiny

Elke Scholz

If not this trail,
which trail?

If not these woods,
which forest?

Crystal lace frames
a frozen palace
secrets rushing under
icy blankets,
to the end or
to the source?

If not these waterfalls,
which waterfalls?

Uncertain dizzy path
pauses in delightful tastes.
Searches falter at crossroads
yearning for a sure fever.
Fog hangs suspended
till sunlight commands evaporation.

Does is all have to matter?

If not this answer,
which answer?

If not you,
then who?

Chikara Warrior Stories

Chikara Warrior Stories and Senjutsu

So many people came up to me after the launch of the Anxiety Warrior Event: learning symposium, April 9, 2017, and book tour, saying that if I could speak, write, and thrive with anxiety, then so could they. It made me realize that with connections and sharing we can encourage and support each other. The following stories are from people that I have met, who have changed their lives despite the challenges they faced. They are Chikara Warriors (Power Warriors) They are thriving. They opened my heart wide, and I am moved to tears of love and admiration when I read their stories and realize that we all have so many different roads to journey. Each one is determined to thrive. It doesn't matter what combination of Senjutsu (tactics) one uses. I hope you find hope, strength, and some ideas from these sharings. Gambaru.

— Elke

A Different Kind of Warrior Now

Kathryn Boland

I've always been a warrior. Well, at least for as long as I remember. Always fighting some force or another, or fixing/changing in preparation for a fight to come. From schoolwork to clothing to friendships, there was always something to fight or to fix. It's not that I liked doing those things. Well, maybe I liked the outcome when it was in my favour. I think that I didn't know how not to fight or to fix.

I remember hearing my big brother Matt (one of three) tell my therapist—me sitting right there—that I used to be a really fun, smiley, and light-hearted kid. And something had really, really changed. Matt was there at his own request; as a practicing clinician himself, he thought he could combine the clinical and familial to create useful insight.

I saw later that the session was useful, but at the time I really wanted to be anywhere else. I sat on that couch, halfway about to cry and halfway wanting to squirm out of my skin. Just as in every one of these sessions, I wanted to leap, sway, lunge, and fall to the floor with my emotions. I was slowly learning then, at the start of a year-long process, that my pain and confusion were rooted in times before my memory could fish them out.

I'm a heady person, so traditional psychotherapy helped me to reason through—and reason out of—faulty thought patterns. But even more so, my anxiety and sadness were caught deep in my body. In my bones. In my muscles. In my fascia. In the face that had a door slammed right into it by bully girls I called my "friends." In the ears that heard the vicious gossip of insecure pre-teen girls, seeing me (likely unconsciously) as an easy target to take down in order to build themselves up.

Most significantly, my parents' separation, and subsequent divorce, truly shook my foundations. It was a rocky period from ages three to seven years old, one that I think that pulled out from under me my very foundations of trust and understanding in the world.

I was also going through a certain level of medical trauma, being diagnosed with a growth hormone deficiency and undergoing subsequent treatment. At seven years old, I had to prick myself with a needle every night (aided by an "Injector" that made it swift and painless, but still not exactly fun).

Born into a white upper-middle-class family, I fully acknowledge my privilege. I am incredibly grateful that my family was able to afford health insurance for this treatment and, as far as pediatric medical treatment goes, it really could have been worse. But I think that these things did set in me a desire to fix or to fight. Never was there pause to breathe, think about the situation, and perhaps call on others for help. I became fiercely independent. I was always going to fix or fight by myself. "No, please don't help," was my attitude.

As an outlet for some of this fierce independence, I became what some might call a tomboy, exploring trails near our house, swimming, sailing, playing soccer. Perhaps the girliest thing I did was riding horses. My first contact with formalized dance education was in a "creative" dance class at a young age. Despite the title, and apparent purpose, I'm told I was yelled at for not following class instructions. All I know is that I didn't formally dance again until age 13. I had become interested in music and theater (I can't recall how or why), and through that found dance. Perhaps it was a part of the re-shaping; defining and truly owning one's identity as a teenager. Perhaps that in dancing, I could fight or fix, and sometimes channel that energy into fleeing, at different times. The only hard part was that I had to do that how and when dance teachers told me to. I've always enjoyed improvising rather than dancing set choreography. But striving for an ideal, and moving with and among members of a group, have their own special power as well.

I danced all throughout high school, and knew that I needed to keep doing it in college. I majored in Dance (along with theater, English and art history minors) at the George Washington University (GWU) in Washington, DC. There I was introduced to totally different ways of thinking about, discussing, feeling, and creating movement, from the Feldenkrais Method to Laban Movement Analysis to postmodern dance methods such as Release Technique.

Partly by being a young adult, partly by the political activism all around me, I was developing a strong socio-political conscience. My drive to use movement for the healing and empowerment of others was blooming. I was also introduced to yoga at this time. There were free classes at GWU's gym on certain weeks, and I had heard it was good cross-training for dancers, so I thought I'd give it a shot. The first class was difficult—maybe even painful in some ways—but something in me was hooked. I kept going back.

At the same time, part of me was deeply hurting and sick. I had my second bout of an eating disorder in my sophomore year. Such disorders are often a symptom of a larger problem. I was often anxious, and was sensitive to the slightest distance between myself and anyone I interacted with. Beneath all of that was a deep sadness, a void. Maybe the anxiety was an unconscious attempt to fill the void. Maybe if I moved quickly enough, maybe if I got enough done, then I could jump right over that void. That didn't quite work; sometimes I fell right in.

But the years progressed, and by the time I graduated I was in a much more settled, healthy place. Yoga, as well the wonderful dance community in which I was engaged, helped me learn to accept myself. I began to eat enough to supply my active body's needs, and I returned to a much healthier weight. Yet there was a new anxiety surfacing; it was clear that a choreographic and/or performance career wasn't in the cards for me. What career could I pursue that would be economically viable, yet satisfy my soul's need to be in movement with others?

I thought of yoga instruction, but something felt untenable and unstable about it. I learned about dance/movement therapy, and as soon as I watched a few YouTube clips of the work I knew this was it. Before I could enter a program, however, I needed undergraduate psychology credits. I moved back into my mother's home, and stayed there for the hardest year and a half of my life. I felt as if I were regressing instead of moving forward, and I didn't react well. The height of it was having two panic attacks, the only I've ever had, in the same weekend.

My anxiety reared its ugly head, a deep sadness—I learned later—underlying it. My mother insisted that I get professional help. It was medication first, then psychotherapy. That's how I ended up on a couch that day with my brother, us both facing my therapist. How I felt then, crawling in my skin and just needing to move, was part of the inspiration I had through a difficult three years of graduate school in dance/movement therapy.

I wanted to offer to people just like me the chance to satisfy that urge, ultimately working towards healing. I got my acceptance letter to Lesley's MA program in the discipline on Christmas Eve of 2011. What a Christmas present! My anxiety story didn't stop there, however. Through graduate school I was strapped for time and money, more than I ever had been before. There was also the pain of facing my demons. After one class watching a video about eating disorders, for instance, I had a panicked outburst at my roommate.

I realized that it was the first time that I had ever accepted the fact of my history with the disorder (I had actually never been formally diagnosed). This is the inner work that helping professionals must do in order to be fully present for those we serve. Through my internships I was beginning that work for others. I had to fully face what I had not yet been present within myself: what needed healing, what I needed to come to accept.

At the same time, I was offering movement and helping to cultivate greater connection to the body for those with memory disorders, then to at-risk youth at an early childhood program. I continued to practice and teach yoga, though at a greatly reduced capacity. And my heart kept calling me back to it. After graduating, facing the stressors of finding work in the mental health field, a very difficult first employment experience, and more full understanding of the rigours and complexities of professional mental health licensing, I decided to return to yoga.

I would teach full-time. This would be my chosen path, my life's work. I haven't left that path since. I still experience anxiety and the sadness that underlies it. Yet I work through it with conscious reflection and my movement/posture practice. I can then be in a place to help others face, and then work at, dissolving their own anxiety. So much of it manifests in the body. Just look at the language we have for anxiety and fear: "sick to my stomach with worry," "pit in my stomach," "chills down my spine," "don't sweat it," "don't sweat the small stuff."

The body can show the present condition of the mind and spirit, but all these parts are even more closely linked than that. Modern science is getting closer all the time to catching up with ancient wisdom in recognizing the inextricable, inseparable nature of the mind/body connection. We're more clearly understanding all the time how and why confining the body to cubicles, car seats, and couches—without opportunity to move, express, and create—so deeply confines the mind and soul.

Conversely, we see and more fully understand that when the body can more often exercise its capacities, it can begin to heal itself, and the mind and spirit. I'll share a few stories of how I've used movement to work towards those goals. In many cases, there's no replacement for conventional and professional medical and/or psychological treatment. In all cases, engaging with the body can help the body, mind, and spirit achieve more of their potential to self-heal.

Veterans

For four years, I have done expressive movement groups at a veterans' homeless shelter; specifically, with those age 65 and older or disabled, as others are encouraged to go out during the day to look for jobs and otherwise be productively active. I start groups with a check in, asking how they've been and if they have any news, such as developments in their housing searches.

Sometimes this turns into a venting session for one or two group members, but what is nice about these times is how the other veterans truly show up for each other in support—no soldier left behind. We share practical advice, empathize, and simply listen. All of this can powerfully chip away at the anxiety and sadness that they often experience.

We then do about 20 minutes of gentle movement and stretching, some of it inspired by chair yoga, some my own movement creations. It's always a fun challenge for me to adapt class content to the veterans' needs: some have significant physical limitations and medical conditions for which even the gentle chair-adapted sequences are not suitable. My goal with these modifications is always to make the veterans feel successful, empowered, and capable.

They've lost a lot—sometimes brothers in battle, sometimes family members. Ultimately, all—despite their service to their country—have lost their homes. Through moving all parts of their bodies, gently back-bending, side-bending, folding forward, rolling wrists and ankles, and more, I can help remind them of what, in their very bodies, is still very much theirs: how they are still whole.

I can see that they are experiencing these truths cognitively, as well as in the body, using guided imagery (such as imagining a favourite place, or a wonderful place in their imaginations). Sometimes I guide them to just follow the sound of their breathing, and notice how they feel after moving in a gentle and balanced way. As I offer closing words, I smile a little and ask how they feel.

They offer short-and-sweet answers like "good," "great," or simply a smile, nod, and "Thank you." Most often someone asks me when I'll be back. In those short movement sessions, the systems of their minds, bodies and spirits get a taste of what it's like to be more connected, integrated, and balanced, and they want more. Surely, for those who have risked their lives for the safety and security of their country, for the upholding of its strongest and truest values, it is the least we can offer these intrepid warriors.

On the pediatric floor

I have also led movement groups—expressive movement, yoga, or some blend as appears best for the participants at hand—at a local pediatric centre. This unit was created specifically for children with chronic or significant care needs, with living areas nearby for families to stay on a short-term basis. Sometimes these sessions were with whole families, and sometimes with one or two parents. Just as with the veterans' groups, I would tailor the movement content according to the needs and desires of the participants.

The energy could be drastically different: a gentle, quiet yoga session with a sole mother, to laughter-filled movement games with a whole family. The only important thing was that all involved came out feeling more connected to themselves in body, mind, and spirit, and perhaps able to shake off some of the weight on their shoulders. A family coping with a child's serious illness is coping with so much: the child with the burden of disease; the parents and siblings with the worry and pain of seeing their flesh-in-blood in pain, and maybe at risk of dying.

It is the medical care that will do the heavy lifting of healing, no doubt, however, expressive movement can process and make the heartbreaking, arduous process a bit more bearable.

"Mind over matter" really means something. This is corroborated by studies on the placebo effect, and by investigations in neuroscience.

The human will to be alive and thrive is strong. Expressive movement and stretching re-kindle that flame. Bringing oxygenated blood to various parts of the body through conscious breath and movement, and all the while having *fun*, is a powerful aid in healing the body.

Allie the Anxious

Allie (as I'll call her for the sake of confidentiality) has been my private yoga student for two years. She wanted to begin sessions because of low-back pain and shooting pains through her shoulders and neck. She is a public bus driver by profession, and the prolonged sitting, with much repetitive movement, has taken a toll on her physical health. We came to find that there was a lot that mindful movement and breath could help her with.

She sees a counsellor, from whom she received a psychological evaluation. She informed me that she was labeled "fight or flight," very prone to act defensively before she might need to. It's not hard to see this in even a few minutes with her, on certain days. She speaks quickly, eyes wide open, and her body appears ready to pounce or run. This has gotten better with our sessions; she seems more able to pause, breathe deeply, and slow herself down. It seems as if we are beginning to unravel hard-wired patterns that were wrapped around and around, over and over, throughout her lifetime.

During our sessions, as we move, stretch and pause for deeper breath, her whole person can seem overtaken with the experience. Her eyes can grow wide, not in the anxious way they sometimes do, but as if her body, mind, and spirit are flooded with the positive power of what is happening for her.

I integrate yogic truths, such as accepting one's self and balancing work and rest, and she sometimes chuckles and adds a comment, sometimes gives an "mmhmm," and sometimes simply breathes (listening, I assume). Thus, body and mind are involved, and the spirit through the transcendent experience of it all.

As we end our sessions, she thanks me. I can see a new air of calm, balance, and holistic integration of all her parts. She still has far to go in her journey toward all that she can be, but I have seen her more able to handle challenges with composure and acceptance, rather than anger and anxiety. Just as with all of those whom I have served with movement, I have joined them in a battle against the forces that challenge their wholeness.

I'm a different kind of Warrior now. Fighting some of my own challenges still, of course, I am able to use what I've gained in those fights to help others face up to their own. It's an ongoing fight. And I'm ready to keep fighting it.

Anxiety Can Lead You Further

Barb Campbell

Anxiety has come into my life many ways through relationships, work, and aging. My faltering marriage, losing trust, and the shock of loss were all devastating. Workplace bullying. My job and its routines were my sources of confidence. I felt good at work: cat to the lion. Then retirement came and I felt lion to the cat, another loss.

My relationships have never been fairytale stories. Without going into detail, I will tell how I dealt with becoming a single mom with three daughters under the age of 10.

I would come home from work before the kids got home from school. I was at a point of huge loss. I felt empty, sick, alone, and sad. Anxiety set in. I would lie on my bed listening to music, Pachelbel's Canon, no words, over and over, crying and releasing the tension from my body, the magic of the music calmed me to peacefulness. I did that for weeks until I eventually became stronger. Retelling the story now, the emotion is still in my body. Over time it has lessened, but there are still tears. It brings back the sadness of that time.

Then I went to talk to someone, not family or friends, but a psychologist. He listened while I dumped everything, I let it all out; I cried and cried. It felt so good. He said I don't need pills.

I knew that I wasn't going crazy or that I needed medication. Instead, I talked and took his advice. He suggested that I travel, and take my kids. I was petrified. And then I thought, sure, why not? Because he suggested it and encouraged me, I found the strength to go. That helped.

So, I started fresh and began building a new bridge. I flew out West to visit my sister and let it all go. It helped me to forget the upsets in my life, knowing that I could do it, me, a single mom with three young children. A vacation from my troubles, in a different environment.

You may think you are beaten, but words and help to push but not pushing motivated me.

What was I feeling during the worst of this period? I could not eat, and went from 68 kg (150 lbs.) to 45 kg (100 lbs.) in a few months. I was skinny and sick looking. I put on a good outer front, but inside I lost trust, I cried, I was unhappy, mad, and lonely, and I made poor choices for myself in new relationships, which did not help. I lost trust in men. I may have felt needy, so I picked a man who was younger and from whom I could walk away.

I was suddenly in many situations, including single and anxious, knowing that now I was responsible for myself and my daughters.

I felt my personality changing from mousy to bold. For example, one day I got frustrated with a guy in an apartment parking lot for blaring music and told him off. This was new for me.

Another time, I went to meet a girl who was bullying my daughter and set a boundary; I told her that enough was enough. She stopped harassing my daughter.

Having to shovel snow made me feel sick, mad, and frustrated because I was doing it rather than my ex, the father of my children, who had taken off. Get the picture? It had been hard finding accommodation to rent, because some landlords did not want to rent to single mothers. The shovelling helped in the end to get the frustration out of my mind.

My choice was to fight all this. Don't give up, don't give in.

I began every type of exercise—yoga, stretching, walking... I went to motivational groups and classes, I pushed myself so I would not to be stuck.

I now serve Communion at church. I never thought that I would get up in front in people and have all eyes on me. Are you kidding me? It took all I could do to get up and serve Communion.

I learned to operate a cash register, even though someone thought I could not learn. I ignored the words and the feelings; this became a challenge and I did it.

It was the challenge that made me do it, that gave me fuel and made me feel powerful. I would show her, and I did.

Sometimes anxiety can lead you further.
Sometimes it can trap you.

Seize what works for you.

I had been weak, shy, inadequate, and bone-rack skinny. I became stronger, articulate and confident, thanks to Elke Scholz's book, *Loving Your Life*.* The book took me step by step. I needed powerful words to help me mentally and physically, to strengthen me. I did the exercises. I started to draw and doodle, too. It was the right timing.

Prayers can help, as can going to church, even if you are not religious. Church is a religion and practice and faith. I went away from my faith and came back.

Say the serenity prayer: "God grant me the serenity to accept the things I cannot change, courage to change the things I can, and the wisdom to know the difference."

Adult colouring books, talking, joining small groups for fun things, all help. Let your inner child come out to play!

Today, I surround myself with positive, loving people. If I feel intimidated, sad and miserable, I remove myself from them.

Give of yourself: Tough moments teach us to love.

Challenge moments are the greatest gifts, because they require sacrifice and giving of self.

* *Loving Your Life*, by Elke Scholz, is a bestseller now in its third edition. It presents a fun, practical approach to well-being, containing over 40 creative exercises. A writer for most of her life, Elke has also published articles in national magazines and produced anti-anxiety wellness kits that help employees, youth-at-risk, and seniors manage anxiety and depression.

The Miracle of Pets

Sarah Clifford

Animals are such agreeable friends—they ask no questions, they pass no criticisms.
— George Eliot

I guess you could say that I had a bumpy life growing up. I had parents who loved me and definitely had my fair share of happy and great memories, but bad things do happen. I dealt with bullies throughout my entire school life. I was picked on or alone throughout most of my elementary and high school years. Along with this, I had to live through my parents' rough separation and divorce, which began two weeks before my 10th birthday. Anger, isolation, and being pulled between parents, one of whom was an alcoholic, were what I had to deal with through my early teen years. Also at this period, I began to be sexually assaulted

At the age of 15 I was tired of shutting myself in my room or hiding out in the barn to escape my mom's unhappiness and alcoholism, so I decided to move in with my dad. Life was better, but unfortunately frequent moves and continued loneliness took place for the remainder of my teenage years. I continued to be sexually assaulted on and off until I was 19 while the rest of this was going on.

But I learned from all that hardship and decided that my goal in life was to help people. To help them feel better when they are in times of need. Something that I feel I needed in all those years of being alone. If I could just help one person feel better, mentally or physically, then I was willing to take that route. I became a fully certified paramedic at the age of 21, and have been doing it ever since. I'm proud to say I still love the profession despite the ups and downs.

My career choice has been no walk in the park, especially in the beginning. Already suffering from low self-esteem and lack of confidence, I entered a field that was male dominated and where paramedics were known to "eat their young." I came out of those early years with mental cuts and bruises, but I soldiered on. The next few years brought a mixed bag of feelings from having to deal with more family drama, traumatic calls, work politics, shiftwork, and a close to career-ending back injury that I managed to overcome. Despite these rollercoaster events, those years also brought with them an amazing husband and two beautiful children.

Looking back, I can see why I developed a generalized anxiety disorder. It wasn't until the suicides of first responders skyrocketed and a spotlight was shone on mental health that I was finally able to put a finger on what was going on with me. I decided in a fit of desperation to ask a doctor for medications that would treat my endless worrying, absolute exhaustion, inability to concentrate, and constantly upset stomach. I walked away from that appointment with no medications, but with an answer that would start me down the very long road to better mental health. I had been diagnosed with burnout, which eventually led to an official diagnosis of generalized anxiety disorder, which was worsened by mental trauma caused by my work. I now knew what was wrong, so I could go about making it better.

I'm telling you the dark side of my history so you can understand how animals have saved my life. The struggles of those years could have easily led me down a very bad road, but animals kept me from going off the rails. I always had an animal in my world at some point while growing up. Dogs and horses were a big constant, but when life became busy and I moved frequently, I even got a rat.

I learned from an early age that watching a dog play and romp carefree would help me to feel carefree, and that I could ride away from all my worries when I got on the back of a horse. Simply breathing in the smell of a horse was enough to take me to a world where I had no cares. Even when I moved all over the place, my little rat could ride around in my shirt pocket or in my sleeve and I knew I was never truly alone. When I spoke to the animals or petted them I always felt a little lightness in my chest and in my head that would bring me back to life, if only for a few minutes.

Research has since shown that pet therapy does actually help people. Petting an animal is known to reduce blood pressure instantly, improve cardiovascular health, and is even said to reduce overall physical pain. In addition to these physical benefits, pet therapy helps to lift spirits, decrease feelings of anxiety, isolation and loneliness, encourage communication, and even help children with physical disabilities or who are struggling with learning how to read. The benefits are endless.

When my husband and I bought our first house, we knew we had to get our dream dogs. It wasn't long before we found my black and brown German Shepherd, Bear, closely followed by my husband's brindle Great Dane, Brillow. Those two were special—our first dogs, in our first home. Our children before children, I guess you could say. Bear was my heart, but it wasn't long before I realized that Brillow had an extra-special personality that I knew and hoped could help others. Her mammoth size, kind disposition, unique colouring, and melting brown eyes just seemed to draw people to her. With this in mind, I decided to continue my quest to help people feel better and had her certified as a therapy dog.

I knew I wanted to visit the elderly in my local hospital. I always felt an air of loneliness during the occasional times I walked on the floor to take people to or from appointments. The hospital didn't have a regularly visiting therapy dog, so the fit was perfect. Brillow became a bit of a celebrity there, all 70 kg (155 lbs.) of her. Her kind heart had staff, visitors and patients all wanting a visit. She had patients who were severely depressed or withdrawn, barely smiled, could barely move, or who didn't talk, smiling, moving a hand to touch her, or mumbling quiet words to her, asking for kisses. Just remembering the lives she touched and the change in people I witnessed firsthand brings tears to my eyes as I type. After a year and half I retired Brillow, because I was getting ready to start my own family with real little humans. I still occasionally get asked about Brillow at the hospital even though it's been years since she was there. She was a strong pup and lived to the ripe old age of 10, outliving my faithful Bear by a few years. She was a good dog.

It wasn't until some years later that I decided to venture back into the therapy dog world. It began with a cute, fuzzy puppy that we had got to help keep Bear and Brillow young in their older years. Gordie was more then special right from the beginning. In January 2011 we lost my husband's mother to cancer. It was a hard hit as she had become my substitute mother. One day, while on holidays during the summertime in a little town called Webbwood, we stumbled across an advertisement for Golden Retriever/Border Collie pups in a corner store window. My husband and I had been talking about getting a third dog for the other two, but were still at odds as to what kind. I wanted a Golden Retriever and he wanted a Border Collie. It was fate! We had to go ahead.

We let our daughters choose the dog. The girls were one and three at the time. My husband and I agreed that we would take the dog that was the most patient with them. Under close supervision it came down to a male and a female. We knew we wanted a male and so we ended up with a cute little black and white fuzzball in our back seat, and two very excited kids for the five-hour drive home at the end of our holiday. If all those coincidences weren't enough, we took him home exactly one month from the day of my mother-in-law's birthday, which was also the day we laid her to rest in Webbwood, at a beautiful set of rapids called Gordon Chutes. So now you know how Gordie got his name. I told you he was exceptional from the start.

One day, while taking a patient back to one of the nursing homes, I saw a therapy dog at work and instantly knew that Gordie would be perfect for it. He was four years old by now and fully trained in all levels of obedience. His kind disposition and soul-searching brown eyes seemed to draw out the best in everyone he met. He passed with flying colours his first level of testing to become a therapy dog.

This time around, in thinking of my own kids, I knew I wanted to work with children. Gordie had done such a good job with his first round of testing and evaluations that he was able to complete his child certification in three months. It usually takes over a year. He never stepped a paw out of place.

With all this under our belts, we began reading with kids at our local school. Kids once too nervous to read and stumbling over words grew confident with Gordie as their mentor. Their smiles and laughter at his silly antics while they read still echo in my memory. It really is something to see a child who is normally quiet and reserved come to life with the help of a dog.

The most heart-touching event in our therapy dog work took place in 2016. We had been asked to take part in a children's grief camp. Honoured, I knew Gordie was up for the task and readily agreed. In June we packed up and headed out for a weekend with children who had recently lost loved ones. That weekend was mind altering. There were many tears in those three days, but also many smiles. We saw kids who had been completely shut down slowly come back to life and open up about things they had never talked about, when Gordie came to see them. Children scared of being away from home stopped crying and even began to smile and interact more with their fellow campers. Words cannot describe what I witnessed when Gordie worked his magic. By the end of the weekend, counsellors came up to us in disbelief at the transformation in kids in just two days. Kids they could not reach no matter how the counsellors had tried opened up to Gordie and me after a simple pet or a light hug. There is no doubt in my mind that Gordie changed lives that weekend. He even got a standing ovation at the closing ceremonies.

So can you see now why therapy pets are so important? Not only has research proven the health benefits, but I have witnessed them first hand with Brillow and Gordie. Next time you see your pet or you come in contact with an animal, pay attention to your body as you pet and talk to them. I bet you will catch your mood lightening, your lips curling up in a little smile, and feel tension easing. Once you feel this magic, you will understand how animals have saved not just my life but countless other lives as well.

Work Anxiety

Magdalene Carson

In sharing my experience with work anxiety, let me first define "work" as the activities required to earn one's living or as tasks that must be accomplished for other reasons. In my case, being self-employed and defining and leading everything in my life myself, the issue of work anxiety presents itself in a particular way. I sometimes imagine that if I were working under a boss, where tasks are defined and time is structured, or engaged in a team, where the collective carries the ups and downs, then things would be much easier. But having experienced these situations, I remind myself that the same anxiety can be experienced in different ways in any situation.

Work anxiety presents itself as an amorphous, constant, unfocussed pressure that I feel driven by every waking hour. I often describe it as a pack of wolves stalking me, even though when I turn around I cannot see them, not unlike the bogeyman under the bed. It has been a constant effort to bring this pressure under control, to tame it using different tactics, techniques, and tricks. Over time, I have made a lot of progress, but constant effort is still required.

The first action is always to dissect the amorphous mass of "things that must be done" into priorities and a plan, to put it on paper and forget about worrying. This can help, but it does not dispel the overwhelming pressure.

Sometimes a large part of the anxiety is performance related: will I succeed in the project and get it done on time? Then I remind myself that I have never failed, that I've solved the most difficult problems and met the most difficult timelines, and that I have excellent relations with my clients. I know, consciously, that I will go through this again, but some part of me cannot let go of these fears. The pressure is still there.

Often I must ask myself: Am I going to be driven by all the pressures around me, or am I going to stay in control? Will I allow myself to be overwhelmed by the chorus of voices that want things done, or do I decide what, when, how, and on what terms? I bring to mind the image of myself in the driver's seat of a car filled with back- and front-seat drivers. No way! I decide when, where, how I am making this trip. The thing is: *Either you are controlled or you are in control.* Or another way of thinking about it: *Who will be in control: the horse or the rider?*

Focus is an important issue. Is your mind a blur with all the needs and demands swirling around? The key thing is to decide to work on one thing single-mindedly until it is done. The thing is: *either you are focused or everything is a blur.*

The work that I do is work that I love. It is Good Work. So how can work that I love become such a painful adversary, when in fact it is a source of happiness for myself and for others, not to mention my livelihood? It is helpful to stop and appreciate this reality. I try bringing to mind an orchard where I go forth eagerly to pick fruit in the order and choice that makes me happy. In other words, to transform this image of my work being a burden into the reaping of happiness.

A lot of my anxiety pain is self-created. For example, setting timelines that are far too unrealistic and, to further punish myself, giving quotes based on these tight timelines. Or setting a plan based on a project's proceeding without a single problem, while projects often encounter some unexpected detour. So-called "working very hard" and neglecting self-care by not taking breaks, by not sleeping and nourishing myself adequately, and by working too long hours will also intensify anxiety. I have to be careful that a general feeling of anxiety does not lead me to manufacture more anxiety.

There are many techniques I have learned to employ to decrease work stress. For example, I don't have to respond to every email or request immediately or answer every phone call. Stay in control of your time, I remind myself. Reply and respond when you are ready and according to your own needs and schedule.

While my work is essentially creative, it requires performing complex technical processes as well as financial and bookkeeping tasks. Remembering all the details and steps to take is stressful for anybody. So as to not have to rely on memory and to be able to quickly find files and information, I maintain detailed manuals and cheat sheets, and other tools. I take the same approach to client files and the progress and communications on each project, keeping well-organized records.

The time of day I begin work is important. I love to start my work by 6:00 a.m. If I start my work at 9:00 a.m, I feel as if the day is almost finished, even though this is completely irrational.

One common reaction to work anxiety is to rehearse the work processes over in my head in advance of actually doing the work. This just heightens anxiety and is of no assistance whatsoever when it comes time to actually doing the work. I try to stop this mental rehearsing as soon as it begins by distracting myself with something else.

And sometimes it simply boils down to just jumping in there and doing it. Think about standing on a dock and all that hesitation and reticence before jumping into a beautiful lake for a wonderful swim. I also remind myself of the tough lives of animals and birds living in the wild and all extremes of weather. They get on with their lives and do what they need to do.

One very important resource for me has been, and is, the mindfulness meditations led by Diana Winston, Director of Mindfulness Education at the UCLA (University of California, Los Angeles) Mindful Awareness Research Center.*

My partner was a university professor for many years. There is always a huge stress before going into the lecture hall to teach a room full of students. He calls it "stress," but you could just as well call it anxiety. He told me of one professor who had it so bad that he would vomit before a lecture. Though he was a brilliant academic, he had to give up teaching because he could not get it under control.

My partner has developed his own techniques to counter pre-lecture stress. For 10 minutes before a class, he sits and does nothing. Does not think about the lecture he will give or the classroom and students. He focuses on a point on the wall. Or he closes his eyes and focuses on a point in his forehead. Focus is the key thing for him: to focus on the content of the lecture.

When feeling like this at other times, he says it is important to try to pinpoint the cause of the stress/anxiety and to ask questions: Why am I so confused? Am I tired? Why am I fidgeting? Where does it not feel good in my body? Do I need water? Do I need a break? Do I need a catnap? Do I just need to close my eyes for a few minutes?

Interestingly, my partner speaks of "stress," not "anxiety," because he is not a naturally anxious person, but I think the same principles apply. His view is that stress is an energy and it is good. It is a big force in life. It gives us impetus and drive, and the strength and power to accomplish what we need to. The issue is to get in control of it, to use it as a positive force, a tool.

Sometimes life surprises you with its lessons. Earlier this year, my father passed away. There was a lot of family time for several months and my work fell behind. However, despite the backlog of work to catch up on, I felt absolutely no anxiety about my work at all. I marvelled at the phenomenon. I wondered if perhaps it was because I was giving myself permission to take the personal time I needed. Then a friend offered a brilliant insight: You have experienced the worst that can happen. We have all heard that advice: If you are overwhelmed with worry, stress, anxiety, or panic, think of the very worst that could happen, so as to put your difficult moment in a realistic perspective. Life seems to have done that for me.

For some of us, mastering anxiety is a long and winding road requiring a conscious approach and new tactics at every bend. I feel that I have made a lot of progress over time, but it is never really gone—yet. This is my latest tactic: I found a little figurine of an ugly, angry goblin and perched him on a shelf overlooking me as I work. I drew an "A" on his breastplate. He makes me smile and reminds me that most of my angst and fears are no more based in reality than this fantastic, scary creature.

* Anyone can listen to these meditations, without cost, at http://marc. ucla.edu/meditation-at-the-hammer.

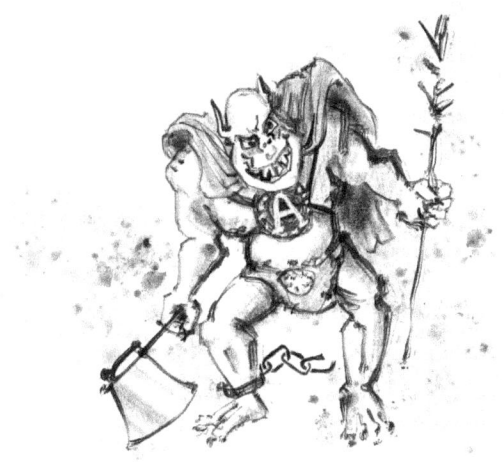

A Moment Can Change a Life

Angie Davis

I had one of those moments, in July 2012, when I was 33. I had a fall. A bad one. From standing, I fell forward onto my face. When I was rolled over, there was no pulse.

There are indents in my floor from where my teeth hit it. I have amnesia about the actual incident and for six hours afterwards. I only know what happened following my fall from second-hand accounts. This is perhaps for the best, not to be able to remember the impact, the pain, the teeth and blood everywhere, the distress of my now ex-partner, and the series of mishaps and mistakes at the hospital.

I know that I was joking with the ambulance attendants at my home, two teeth on the floor, a third shoved up into my upper jaw bone, a fourth shattered in half and dangling from my mouth. I know I said over and over again, hundreds of times that night, "What happened? What happened?" I know my CAT scan test was clear. I know one of the first fuzzy memories from when my brain started coming back on board is of me sobbing, "My teeth, my teeth." I suspect the loss of them was the only concrete thing to grasp onto in a time of utter confusion and shock. I know I was sent home several hours later with zero follow-up care and zero information on concussions. At home that morning, I urinated in the bed and could barely be woken up. This, too, was part of my trauma.

The bones in my upper palate were broken and I eventually lost four teeth. I wore a denture for several years while dental surgeries healed, and hundreds of hours in a dental chair resulted in a new smile. Exceptional dental care from the dental surgeon and my dentist is one stroke of positivity on my healing path. It took a year to get the bones in my skull back into place and to heal my intensely painful whiplash injury. I had tried to stop myself when I fell, but I fell so fast it didn't matter. I have a wrist sprain that was only recently discovered and is still healing.

But I also sustained invisible injuries to my brain from my head hitting the floor. The human head weighs around 4.5 kg (10 lbs.), and when it falls even from a mere 1.6 metre (5'3") height a lot of damage can ensue. Thank goodness I am not taller.

While the physical injuries were painful and extensive, living through a brain injury was life and soul altering. If you imagine the parts of my life as various shades of coloured glass bottles, in the same moment that my head hit the floor, it was as if someone holding these bottles dropped them all and my life broke into thousands of pieces, just as the bones in my face shattered like corn flakes crumpled in your hand.

For over two years, "I" was lost to mild traumatic brain injury. I went from being an active triathlete and dedicated teacher to being unable to read, remember details, or organize my life. Because of the lack of medical care, I returned to work as an elementary school teacher much too soon. I had no one to tell me otherwise, and didn't realize the extent to which my own thinking and self-reflection were impaired.

The lights, the noise, the cognitive load of thinking and problem solving, the multi-tasking demands of my career, these were all impossible to manage. During every single break, I went into a small, dark room, put in ear plugs, turned out the lights, and lay down with something over my eyes. Three to five times a day I did this. After work is a blur, but I know there was a lot of discomfort, a lot of isolating myself to bear the intense queasiness and pain.

My headaches were so bad I took eight Tylenol a day for months. I was initially told my body could process this much, but when I was finally able to see a neurologist five months after the fall I was told that consuming this much pain medication was actually harmful and would likely cause even more rebound headaches.

For months I could not sleep. The fatigue was so all-consuming that many times I ended up going to work in jogging pants, without having brushed my hair. I simply did not have the cognitive ability to say, "I cannot do this."

Five years later, I am still gathering all those glass pieces and pasting them together to make a new image, a new life. The big, overall loss was my sense of safety and trust in my own body. But there are layers upon layers of other losses: teeth, my self-identity, time, trust in the medical system, faith in those closest me to get me help, marriage, extended family, friendships, and more.

It took me years to gain enough mental and physical strength to be my own advocate. Brain injury is often called the invisible injury as people can't see the hurt and the damage, which instead comes out through words, behaviours and actions. But for me, I look at pictures of myself for the entire two years and see only physical evidence of suffering. It was in my eyes: crossed, small, vacant, suffering, unsmiling, dead eyes.

When I was healthy and strong enough to start asking questions— "How did this happen to me? Why didn't you see? Why didn't you get me help?"—the answers were equally devastating. "All head injuries are different," from the doctor. "I was just trying to survive too," from my husband. "I don't know how this happened to you," from the neurologist. There were no answers anywhere, only me being left not knowing how I was so very badly missed by the systems and people that were supposed to protect and support me when I couldn't take care of myself.

I will also never know if I lost my marriage because I had a brain injury and it was too hard, or because I had a brain injury and my partner had no one to help him understand me, to help him see that despite my impaired words and actions, I was fighting hard to not only heal but also to simply see and make sense of the shattered pieces on the floor.

Becoming clear about and integrating these layers of loss takes time and courage to feel the intense anger, bloody outrage and consuming sadness and grief.

I still don't know why my body gave out on me and if or when it may happen again. I have no diagnosable blood pressure, heart, or vitamin or mineral issues. My fall was not considered fainting as people who faint feel woozy, see stars and crumple, instead of falling flat on their faces like I did. My fall was more like a seizure, but all medical tests indicate a body and brain in good health. Not knowing why has been impossible to live with. My brain has actually adopted interesting strategies to cope with the lack of a concrete answer.

The thoughts of another fall, of all that damage happening again, of the potential for disability or death if it happens again, cause feelings of terror, panic, and anxiety. I have been diagnosed with posttraumatic stress disorder (PTSD). PTSD is an anxiety disorder, one which I personally liken to anxiety on the most potent and powerful steroids you can find.

My PTSD symptoms have gone through many incarnations in five years. For two and a half years after the fall, there were long periods of time when I was afraid of everything and everyone, when even little daily stresses left me shaking in extreme fear, as if my entire life itself were at risk. Cumulatively, the weight of the fear often sent me hiding under the covers or into a closet. I spent hours, days, weeks in my bed. Sometimes I would feel so reactive and unsafe in the world, with the knowledge that a fall could happen at any time, that I would hide in closets. I lived in constant fear. Would I hurt someone? Would I die? Would I lose the teeth we worked so hard to repair? The closed-in space provided the only semblance of safety I could feel.

I used to be ashamed of and judgmental towards these coping behaviours. Why wasn't I stronger? Why couldn't I do something else? Why couldn't I emerge and just communicate? But I have since learned to have more compassion for that hurting version of me: I did the best that I knew how. I understand that I had a true traumatic reaction and used whatever coping strategies I had available to help me feel safe. I now choose to see that the woman hiding under the covers, seeking safety in closets, was fighting for her life.

It was actually after one of these closet-hiding episodes that I emerged with a sense that I needed to do something different. And so began a journey learning about my anxious, traumatized brain, how to understand it, help it, have compassion for it, and support it along a healthier path.

This journey means directly addressing my PTSD triggers and anxiety-inducing thoughts and behaviours. I work with a "body-based" therapist, who is helping me rebuild the relationship between my mind, brain, and body. My therapist also practices eye movement and de-sensitization reprocessing therapy EMDR. My current largest, panic-inducing triggers include having to talk about my fall, and any talk or mention of death or head injury in conversations, books, television, and/or movies. I am also working to sense and feel my face again, as my traumatic reaction cut off this sensation. This involves working with the smashed-in, broken-boned skeleton face that visits me in the dark, a reminder from an anxious brain to remember and be afraid.

But I am learning instead to befriend all of these images and symptoms as messengers, each piece giving me a little bit of information about how my brain and body are doing, and what is begging to be seen and worked with (usually, for me, fear). I am slowly developing the belief and faith that I have the strength and the resources to greet these messengers, listen to them, hold space for their fears, and respond to them in a meaningful way. Each time I sit with them, their strength and impact are softer. It is like sifting through broken pieces of coloured glass, finding one to hold up to the light, turning it over and over until I recognize its curves and edges, the way it feels in my hand, its dimples and imperfections. And only then can I add this piece to the new stained glass artwork taking shape.

Recently I was asked, "What didn't break?" My immediate answer was, "One thing. The light I am. My essence." It has been important for me to realize that in this respect I am lucky. Sometimes, the traumatic reaction is so complete that a person feels their light has gone out.

Many things have helped me re-integrate my sense of self. Yoga practices such as sensing my breath and my body have helped me feel my body again. A practice called iRest, which is a modern adaptation of the ancient practice of yoga nidra*, has helped me calm my body and mind over time. Putting many small self-care strategies front and centre on my daily agenda helps me manage my anxiety in a preventive way, teaching me to be aware of my mental, emotional, and physical states so I can address any imbalances as soon as possible. Physical exercise, having a few close friends who offer endless amounts of patience and support, and seeking therapy have also all helped me gain strength, recover, and learn about my new needs. As I do the work of unlocking the trauma, I feel lighter and lighter, and the path ahead of me is becoming more and more clear. I am now profoundly grateful to still be on this Earth, to be able to breathe and move and feel and connect.

I believe I survived so that I can help be the light for other people. This pull to have my story be of service is starting to change my life. Things are aligning in my different roles in the world. I have become a yoga teacher and am supporting people to come home to themselves by understanding their minds and feeling their bodies. I have aspirations to support those on their own medical and emotional healing journeys. In my career, I am working with mental health initiatives and have become passionate about helping students and my fellow educators understand the silent struggles that trauma, anxiety, depression, oppression, and more impose on the brain and on our ability to learn.

The passion and the purpose came out of the pain. I couldn't have one without the other. In this way, I am able to see my fall and ensuing physical and emotional journey for the gifts they have given me and the positive ways they have changed my way of being in the world. I am a more open, aware, and empathetic person. I understand the darkness and the light, the pain and struggle as well as the triumph and joy, and bring this insight into my encounters. My journey has taught me self-understanding and self-care, returning me over and over again to the things I need for true happiness: nature, writing, yoga, exercise, adventure, and connection. I will never be the same person as before my fall, and thank goodness for that because the world needs cracked-open Angie.

Today, and every day, may you take one step closer to your own healing and health.

* Yoga nidra is among the deepest possible states of relaxation that one can achieve while still maintaining full consciousness. It has been described as a state of consciousness between waking and sleeping in which the body is completely relaxed, and one becomes increasingly aware of the inner world by following a set of verbal instructions. See resources in Angie's chapter (page 138).

I'll Be Fine

Amanda Duncan

I'm sure you've all had a challenge or two in your days. Imagine a wild animal like a bear right in front of you. First thing, you have to get the hell out of there and survive. For me, having cancer was like that.

Yep, I was a typically healthy 33-year-old and I had cancer. I was diagnosed with a rare aggressive from of cervical cancer that had metastasized to my lymph nodes.

It began in November 2011, following a routine Pap test. The result was normal, okie dokie, A+. Then, in March 2012, I was required to have my IUD out, which came with a courtesy Pap test. Little did I realize that would be the beginning of it all. But I'll be fine, I told myself.

The test revealed high-grade precancerous cells. You then have to wait three months before testing again to see if things change or grow. But I'll be fine, I told myself again. I started to hold my breath more now.

June 2012: After my 12-hour night shift at the hospital and the morning of my mother's open heart surgery, I stopped by the hospital for a quick colposcopy.* Could I think about this now? Not a chance. I stashed that one away for later. My mother, age 54, was on her way in for a quadruple bypass. I thought, *I'm not going to be selfish and think of me, my family needs me. I'll be fine.*

The colposcopy didn't go so well. My gynecologist noted two spots of high-grade cancer cells located on my cervix. I had a Loop Electro-surgical Excision Procedure (LEEP) done in September (in this procedure a low-voltage electric current delivered by a fine wire is used to remove abnormal tissue). The tissue was then sent away to Pathology for a detailed review. "I'm sure it's fine," I would tell myself again. "I'll start going to yoga, relax myself!" My neighbour Mel had a private yoga studio in her home, and I felt so at ease attending her classes.

In October 2012 the results came in. I was always told, "Don't worry, no news is good news." It was then that I was accidentally diagnosed with cancer. I had chipped a tooth on a frozen treat and booked an emergency dental appointment. In addition, I felt like I was getting a urinary tract infection (UTI), so as I was in the same town as my doctor, I thought I'd better see him, too.

Without an appointment I sat in that waiting room with my spouse for four and a half hours. Our tension levels began to rise. I had little patience for his frustration with waiting, as I, too, had building frustration. I mean, who gets up in the morning and looks forward to an emergency dental visit?

I finally told Noel, "Go sit in the car and play on your iPod, I'm sure it's not long now." So he went to the car for some fresh air and waited. I was called into the room just then. The doctor came in with wind behind him and said, "Oh good, I needed to speak with you." I quickly said, "Okay? I think I have a UTI." He then said, "We'll deal with that in a minute."

He sat on his stool looking at his chart, then looked up at me and said, "I don't know how to tell you this, but you have cancer."

My heart sank and a ball of who knows what stuck in my throat. All my brain was telling me was... "You have a UTI."

He read out the results and as much as I listened, I don't know what he said. I can recall his body language, tone, and the lead-up, but nothing more. I was present for that part, so why couldn't I absorb it? Then off to my emergency dental appointment to fix a broken tooth. That was hard. Lying there while someone was fixing my tooth for an hour and all I wanted to do was cry in my husband's arms.

Unknown stage, unknown grade, unknown outcome. What next? The waiting game had just begun. I know everyone has lived through what they felt was an impossible wait at least once in their life. The thought of waiting to find out if you have the chance to live or are, quite frankly, dying... Well, just thinking of that moment I feel tightness in my chest and tingling tears welling. This feeling would continue in the days, weeks, and months that followed. I like to think I am good at compartmentalizing. I can put all the thoughts I want in a bag and leave it at the door, but this was like a cargo ship both in quantity of thoughts and the weight I felt I was carrying around every moment of every day.

In one particular yoga session I began to cry during the relaxing part, and after that I slowly stopped going. Why though, since I enjoyed it? I worried I would disrupt others and was upset that I was so distracted with my looping thoughts.

Three weeks after the LEEP was done, I started calling my gynecologist once a week. For two of those weeks the results sat in a pile on the secretary's desk. Then the gynecologist called me in. I knew he meant business when he said, "This is what I can do, but I think you should see someone at Princess Margaret Hospital (in Toronto) for a second opinion." In my books, this man was one of the best. Still, unknown stage, unknown grade, unknown outcome.

I noticed I had an aversion to saying I would be fine, so now I didn't. Little did I know that I was creating a boundary for my brain and teaching it a new trick. A good one? Nope.

I found a quote on line that said, "You never know how strong you are until being strong is the only choice."

I took that as my goal and ran with it. I mean, I had a six-year-old son, a great husband, and I was in the last year of college for the Practical Nursing program, part time. I worked two jobs as a personal support worker, one at a long-term-care home and one at the hospital. What was I going to do? Curl up in a blanket and hide away in the closet? I thought of that. Sure, it would be cozy, but in the small house we owned at the time we only had one closet and it was already too full. I had no choice. Getting through it was all I had to choose from.

Just a wee bit of stress on my plate. I didn't party or have many friends. Whom would I talk to about this? My dearest friend Shay lived five hours away, and I knew it would make her feel so bad she would feel she needed to come. So, I didn't call her either. I didn't want to upset my husband by making him sad, or our parents and family. Besides, did I really want to be a downer? Nope, not me.

So I didn't talk to them about it.

I was a patient watcher on many shifts at the hospital during this time of figuring out my cancer. It was surprisingly difficult to not think about the impending doom that might be the end of me and my life as I knew it. Did I show my love to others enough? Did I let them know how much I appreciated them?

I would go into a tailspin and feel sicker than when I started. Some of the physical symptoms I had were heartburn, indigestion, and insomnia. I couldn't focus and would get distracted easily. "Burny belly" followed me everywhere, which made me feel nauseous 24/7. I did not realize that I was experiencing physical signs of anxiety.

You may be wondering what I did about it. Well, nothing at the time. I kept going to work and trying my best. I had this idea that my coworkers maybe were not impressed with me leaving early or taking time off, but it was all I could do to get up in the morning and even partially carry on. I would go to school and push through the days of excited student mode, and the ups and downs of life.

Then it happened. They called me in for a Computed Tomography (CT) scan and a Magnetic Resonance Imaging (MRI) scan. Not only was I going home upset and sick here and there; and taking extra days off sick, but now I had to go for a CT scan on Christmas Eve and an MRI on Dec 27. Our li'l family tradition was going to Uncle Tom's restaurant on Christmas Eve. We'd celebrate with family and friends with food, have fun with the children, and taper off with a read-aloud children's Christmas story. December 27, well, that was my father-in-law's birthday. "Great, I'm going to leave my six-year-old son with you to busy up your day, and take your son to Toronto for my selfish supporting needs."

I was scheduled to work both days at the hospital, but they kindly gave me the time away despite how it may have looked. Wait a minute, why am I worried about how it looks? I have cancer for goodness' sake?! Learned behaviour.

February 28: I had my surgery and was told by the surgeon, "It was more invasive then we expected, but I got it all." I was told to come back in two weeks for a follow-up, and someone would call with an appointment date. Three weeks went by and no one called, so I did. I arranged an appointment for the next week. I went in the exam room and was given a lovely blue gown to put on. I got dressed and then the doctor came in to find me lying on the exam table. He right away said, "I don't think we need to do that right now. Did you come alone?" I felt my inquisitive side wake up. "Yes," I said.

He told me to get dressed and he would be back in a moment. I changed my clothes and placed my cell phone on audio record. The next two hours felt like an instant.

He told me that after reviewing the frozen segments removed for pathology, they found cancer cells in my lymph node. The conversation continued with the doctor saying that I was the eighth case like this that he had dealt with. It was a rare, aggressive cervical cancer that had metastasized and jumped to my lymph nodes, rather than spreading to a more typical area.

I could hardly breathe. A parade of specialists came into the examination room to talk to me about options. I just wanted one of them to tell me what to do. Instead, they listed the choices. I had to decide alone. A nurse came in to provide support, but I was dumbfounded. How could I make a decision right now? What if I chose the wrong treatment?

Ultimately I chose the chemotherapy—kill everything in my body and hope the terrible saying isn't true: "If the cancer doesn't kill you the chemo will." No pressure. After the appointment I made the two-hour drive from the cancer centre alone. I called my mom, my sister-in-law and a friend on the drive as I couldn't bear the silence and the noise of my own thoughts.

Seven months of treatment and school kept me anxious and busy. Stress was a part of me every day. I found that gardening was a lovely way to relax. Looking forward to healthy fruit and vegetables was a staple each day and became fun for our family. Three weeks after my treatment ended, I was fortunate to participate in the Terry Fox run on a bike with my son and husband. When I saw a sign at the five km mark that said, "I run for my mom," I began to cry. I was proud to be there with my guys, and alive.

Follow-ups every three months for the first two years kept my worries fuelled and my thoughts looping. It was then that I realized I wasn't fine. All I was focused on was getting through the thick of it, but in the end, I crashed.

On a scale of zero to 10, where zero is no tolerance and 10 is lots of tolerance, my tolerance was about a one out of 10. My emotions where shutting down. I become a pro at raising my voice and was learning the knack of being angry for no reason.

That was the point when Elke came into my life. At the time, I didn't know how positively she would change my life. I was referred to her after I called my workplace Employee Assistant Program. Elke, as I soon learned, has many credentials and they are very fancy but to those I know, I refer to her as "my Life coach." During just a few short visits with her she told me I was experiencing signs of anxiety and had post traumatic stress related to my cancer.

She taught me some tools:

> ✦ Through guided imagery I now have a box that houses
>   my anxious feelings. It's not locked and sits in my
>   imaginary green house with a red comfy chair. The
>   healthy, anxious feelings I sometimes need can still

get out, but only when I want them to and I can visit anytime I like.

✦ I realized that not everybody can see me where I am, and that is okay. We don't all have to be the same.

✦ I have a "junk journal" where I started to write my worries down every day at the same time. I quickly realized I didn't want to worry and it only lasted three days. I know it's there if I need it, though.

✦ I keep a little bottle of lavender water on my desk and when I get worked up or stressed I just put a little on or take a deep breath and enjoy the lovely scent.

With my emotions going up and down, I learned that I can use my own energy shield to keep the things I don't want near me, from me.

I am still learning more tools, but I am in control of me now. Today, I can say I'll be fine, and I cry from happiness when I do.

Amanda Duncan, RPN, is a coordinator for an assisted living service program for high-risk seniors. She and her husband Noel both write about their journey through her diagnosis and treatment in "A Couple's Experience: His and Her Viewpoints," which follows.

*A medical diagnostic is often recommended if a Pap test has shown abnormal results.

A Couple's Experience:
His and Her Viewpoints

Amanda and Noel Duncan

People say there are many sides to a story, so for this one we thought we would give you his and hers. Who are these people, you might ask? We're just a couple living around the corner, working hard, paying bills, and passing the time as a family. We might look like your neighbour, or the cranky cart-wielding heel grabber in the grocery store, or even like your best friends. We are Him and Her.

He says, "Okay baby, let's talk about our adventure."

She says, "All I can think is that this feels more like a black hole. An adventure is supposed to be fun. Taking about illness and emotions, not so much, I think."

Like everyone else, we both have had our share of anxious moments over day-to-day topics such as being late for work, did I turn off the coffee pot? did I send my son off with enough healthy snacks for lunch? If you asked either of us if we had anxiety, we would have shrugged it off. Neither of us could have clearly expressed how anxiety manifests in some people, other than maybe the more known signs like panic or meltdowns.

To give you a sense of what it was like and how it affected us as a couple, we thought we would look back and write as a couple about when our worries came up close and personal. It's a multi-sided story.

Cancer scare: Him

The moment my wife found out she had precancerous cells I noticed a change in her that was the spark of what would become a life's worth of worries and, hopefully, controlled anxiety. I witnessed a change in her even though she fought as hard as she could to bury the worries.

They were present in her mind at all times. I could feel the anxiety even though we didn't talk about it, even though I was being the husbandly reassuring voice. There was now an elephant in the room.

My introduction to anxiety came out of sympathy and worry, being just plain so upset to see someone you love hiding their own concern for their life. Then, through a natural stage of evolution, her anxiety became my anxiety for her. I wanted everything to be perfect. I wanted the best news from the doctors, and for our lives to continue on in the happy, hopeful way they always had. This wasn't cancer yet, this wasn't terminal news, this was "Oh, we'll just keep our eye on this kind of stuff," but that's all it has to be when it comes to a terrible disease that you have watched take so many loved ones before.

My worries and concerns flowed daily. As strong as you try to be and act as if it's nothing, this certainly introduced me to the world of anxiety in a recognizable form for the first time.

Cancer scare: Her

Let's be honest for a minute here. As the "her" in this context I don't even know what to say. If you asked me at the beginning, when I found out I had cancer, I would have told you "I'm fine, it's all going to be okay."

How it all started… returning to the car from the doctor, shutting the door behind me, I heard him say, "So, what do you have?" Thinking I likely had a urinary tract infection. I said, "Well, I'll tell you how my doctor told me. I don't know how to tell you this, but I have cancer."

When I review my memory bank I can recall countless, I mean countless moments when others would say, "Just be positive, it's all going to be fine." Come on now, I had the biggest smile and show for everyone, but inside I was withdrawn and isolated. I would talk with others about my diagnosis as if to calm and reassure them, not me. Inside I was a nervous wreck. The doctor had just dropped a bomb on my lap and I'm left with metaphorical shrapnel in every spot on my body.

I didn't want to be the one who said so selfishly, "Why me," but that's what I was thinking. I couldn't understand, why me? I was a hard-working mom of a six-year-old boy, a very domestic wife, and a college student. The more I think about "why me" versus "why someone else," I couldn't answer that either. It would be terrible, horrible, if it were anyone else, so I would never think it should be on someone else, so it should be me, I would tell myself. Why shouldn't I crawl into my closet or under my covers and cry? I would say to myself, "Just do it! Who says you can't cry yourself to sleep?" So I took the late sleepless nights, the sick days and the constant feelings of unwellness and packed them into myself as if they were mine to guard.

The only thing is that it became my armour, a barrier rather then something I would talk about or deal with. I just accepted the consistent discomfort and would tell myself, "You're okay; it's part of the process, you'll be fine."

We have grown up in a time when society has taught us to think of anxiety as an inconvenience; something awkward. In previous years no one shared how anxiety can manifest in people, unless they went to their doctor and asked, or maybe searched Dr. Google. People were quick to jump rather than look at the bigger picture. You didn't talk about your feelings after school or at the dinner table, like we do now. You didn't even share them at bedtime during a quiet one on one. If you had any "issues," you were to just deal with them, write them in your diary or in a heartbreaking lyrical masterpiece. So if this is how we grew in our society, then what next? The things we feel but don't share, those are the hardest.

Cancer confirmation: Him

The progression from precancerous cells to full-blown cancer in need of treatment brought on an entire new world of fear and concerns. Now the simple old phrase of, "It's going to be fine," or "These days they can take care of this if it's caught early," just didn't seem to work anymore. Once again it was a relit fire in the woman I love, who now had her entire world to fight for.

She had done such a great job of hiding her worries through the initial testing and procedures, but at this moment her level of worry even had me scared. I could feel it across the room. I could see it in her eyes. I could hear it in her voice when she talked.

Every moment of every day in her eyes she could be slipping away. It killed me to watch and try to smile and make her feel better, knowing my words bounced off her and would never make it through, but I still kept throwing them at her and tried to remain positive, reassuring, and hopeful for her. My heart would race, I would have butterflies in my stomach, I would feel sick thinking of what she was going through, most of all thinking about what our son and I could lose. Yet I thought I didn't have any anxieties, I wasn't affected by these feelings, I was just a husband who felt bad for what his wife was going through.

Cancer confirmation: Her

I wasn't sure if I should cry and scream, bearhug my husband and never let go, or curl up into a ball. I stayed strong because I "knew" that was how he needed me to be.

Where do you start? I didn't know how to talk about this. Is it "supposed" to be a casual conversation with, "Okay, so now that I have cancer..." or "Let's make a will."? I became indecisive. What if I make the wrong decision? Let's not forget that my cancer was da da daaa... Cancer down there! Muahahaha!

Nobody talks about that, let alone that part of our body. Maybe it's easy for others, but if you really think about it, it's difficult being intimate when "that's" where cancer is camping out. It's not hiding. it's there burning a bright fire waiting for the next thing/stage. So again, I didn't talk about it. I held it all in. I would talk to others about the cancer. I wanted them to know what to look for. My symptoms came fast and furious and I wanted women, men, everyone to know what to watch out for.

A co-worker of mine was diagnosed with cancer just after me. We had many similar emotions and felt comfortable not having to "bother" our loved ones with our panicked thoughts. Talking together became a great outlet for us, and we would share some of our looming thoughts.

We had sort of open forum discussion/venting sessions during which we would talk and talk. We became great friends, but I continued not sharing my true worried thoughts with my husband. Again, I didn't want to cause him any distress by showing him that I was upset and worrying. The deeper "Who am I" stuff stayed buried inside. I didn't share that with anyone. I just figured that I would find out later. The world will show me who I am when it's good and ready. I still didn't realize at the time that I was crumbling.

Now it's all said and done, I thought. Cancer has reared its ugly head. Time to start our battle! From beginning to end there is no stopping us. These are not the usual day-to-day things we might go through, but it was now.

With our armoury stocked full, the troops lined up in a row, the catapults loaded, we were now poised for battle. You couldn't get more prepared.

Going in strong and full of vigour, how quickly the mighty turned to meek.

Preparing for treatment: Her

Pfft, ya right! He was all like "Roar," and I was all like 'I know I have to do this but how can I? What if I make the wrong decision somewhere along the line or on treatment?'

When I would think about my cancer, whether it was about treatment options, potential outcomes or even just procedures like my peripherally inserted central catheter (PIC line) or the five nuclear medicine injections directly into my vagina while I was awake, it was like a number line-up in my head. It goes like this: I walk up to the round red disc, take a paper number, and then go up to the counter and ta da, done. Next!

Cancer was there; I knew it but I wouldn't go past that. I knew I was upset. I am not denying that. So, it's all good then? Negative.

Preparing for treatment: Him

We were doing this on our terms, as in the treatment wasn't going to take her hair away, we were. So ha-ha cancer, we beat you to it.

We handed our son the electric razor and let him begin the process of shaving her head. As he took the first swoosh I remember feeling extreme concern for how she was going to handle this. She was pulsating with worry, but man did she sit strong.

The first feeling I had when we finished shaving her head was of relief. She looked really good with stubble. I believe the quote was, "You have a really nicely shaped head."

Shortly after that we were on our way to Sunnybrook Health Sciences Centre in Toronto for her first treatment. We had gone through the PIC line insertion and nuclear medicine injections, but this was the first day of chemotherapy. When my wife finally got put into a chair, I can remember my mind jumping, my heart racing, and being completely in a situation of not knowing what to say to the woman I love because I knew nothing I could say would make her feel better. As I held her hand, I watched them hook the lines up to her, give her a brief pep talk, and turn on the chemo infusion pump.

None of these things were "my anxiety," they were just worries for my loved one.

Moments after her chemo began, I went to get a pop and told her everything was going to be okay. I was only gone for a short time. When I returned, the first thing I saw was how flushed her face was. While she was saying she didn't feel right, I watched her go three shades of red. It scared the crap out of me. She was having an anaphylactic reaction to her chemotherapy medication.

It only took the nurse a matter of minutes to stabilize her and find the right additions and flow rate for her treatment. However, the words, "Don't worry hun, you'll be fine," just didn't seem to work after that moment.

Watching her go through the phases of chemo, losing her hair, appetite, and energy, etc., brought on more feelings of worry—for her of course, because I had no anxieties. It was a long process of ups and downs for the next seven months of treatment.

I drove a delivery truck at the time and would spend hours every day alone in the truck wondering how she was feeling and if she was okay. Watching my wife battling for her life while looking so frail was the first moment I thought, my god I could lose her, was it going to be cancer that takes her or the treatment?

During treatment: Her

I remember the doctor saying, "Now if you ask me when you're done treatment if you're going to be okay, I can't say." I felt tightness in my chest and spiralling thoughts. I found myself thinking, "Well, you suck," while also thinking, "He has to be honest, I guess." My learned behaviour would repeat the old saying, "If the cancer doesn't kill them, the chemo will."

I started the treatment terrified, expected the worst but hoped for the best. While going through those seven months I don't know how we did it. My husband was like the captain of an army and I a mere soldier. He stood tall, not appearing to be afraid of anything. Me, I was all suited up but that was about it.

He spent every 12-hour chemotherapy treatment day by my side. While I slept the first three hours from the cocktail of medications they gave me to prevent another anaphylactic reaction, he would sit patiently with the odd giggle to the nurse over my snoring. When I woke, we would talk about mindless stuff or watch TV and just be there together.

Even though I sat there smiling, I wasn't okay. I was devastated.

After each treatment there were some hard days. The fear of not knowing what to expect or if something would be worse or new this time was difficult.

While my husband was at work my six-year-old would help me by getting snacks and reading to me or playing simple games indoors. We would read the book, *Mommy Has Cancer*. Preston would look up at me with his whole heart in his eyes. My husband would carry me the six metres (20′) to the kitchen table for a meal, even though I couldn't eat it.

Makes me teary typing these lines, and there's that lump that shows up in my throat now when I'm sad but tough.

My father would come over on the Fridays after treatment and just be there with me. I would stay focused on my family, studying for exams and working in our garden. The gardening gave me much-needed time outside without having to do too much.

How about just showing up?

My friends didn't come around; they didn't know what to say, but neither did I. "How about just showing up?" but I knew they were busy, I would think. Otherwise, I felt good. I thought, "I can do this. I've got my boys, my guys!"

You never know how strong you are until being strong is the only choice.

Post treatment: Him

So, she got to ring the bell. Through each treatment as we sat with her going through the process, we would hear the faint sound of a bell dinging. The first time I heard it I looked at her, confused. She began to cry as she told me that when you complete your last treatment and your battle is over you ring the bell to signify the healing process has begun.

Each time we heard that bell ring, someone had just completed what they were going through. When it was her turn, I held her hand as we walked down the hallway to the nurses' station where the bell was located. She was gripping my hand more tightly than I thought she had strength to at the time. I'm pretty sure she held her breath the whole way.

She rang that bell and took a deep breath. Walking out of that place, looking at all of the patients waiting for their turn, you feel horrible for what they are all going through, but we were done. This was our turn to breathe.

Through the weeks and months afterwards, I waited every day for a quick return to normalcy. That wait for me, hoping to see the worry shed from my wife, was an emotional process. I would ask her how she felt, and she would say gross. I would tell her she would feel better soon. It was right back to the good old reassuring-husband days—saying what I thought she wanted to hear but never knowing the words that would help. I would get knots in my stomach when I wanted to ask her about it. It was such an emotional topic for her; she didn't want to talk about it.

I think at that time we were both hoping for a miracle because the battle might have been over, but looming ahead were all the "what-if's" and follow-up appointments. Every now and then something would remind us of the next check-up. Instantly the fears came back, as though they had never left. I can remember trying to ignore them and stay focused on whatever we were doing. Trying not to show that I was even thinking about it, but who was I kidding. She was thinking the same thing.

Not wanting to upset each other, we wouldn't talk about it. Hoping it all would go away. For the first time in my life, I was unable to just find a way to put it aside. This brought on feelings of helplessness and inadequacies. It was a long process over the next two years, but with each check-up coming back with good news, my worries slowly started to subside.

Post treatment: Her

So then what? The treatment was done. My husband and I could celebrate and look forward to our next 13 years together. But for me, the next chapter had just begun.

Three years after my first diagnosis, I began to find myself frustrated and angry and quick to judge. I couldn't explain it. Little did I know, but one of the greatest challenges was about to start. Before that moment I think he knew it, but I didn't until that instant.

"I need help," I thought to myself.

So I stood on the stairs in front of him and said, "I think I need to talk to someone professionally." He smiled and hugged me.

Him

Fast forward a year later, she found herself really needing to talk to a counsellor experienced with PTSD patients—people who had gone through hard times and needed help moving forward. She found someone through her work—Elke—and made an appointment.

After the first session she came home elated. Tears of happiness this time. She had found someone who focused on exactly what she was looking for and offered a series of great tips.

It wasn't until that moment that I had ever considered therapy to be of any help. I had to see the change it could bring and the hope it could give. It took seeing hope in her eyes to make me believe that it can help.

I still have apprehensions about therapy because of an unsatisfactory experience I had when I was younger. However, for people who have gone through traumatic situations I now believe it is absolutely necessary in order to help them recover and move forward. It has opened my eyes to a much larger side of the industry and one I think I needed to see first before putting faith in it.

Once I started seeing her practicing the things she learned from Elke, I could see a stronger fight to improve her mental health. It made me so excited to see her addressing this.

It wasn't until this point that I began to recognize that the feelings I had experienced all along were directly related to anxiety. The more I saw what she was going through and having to deal with, the more I realized I, too, was engulfed in the same battle. However, my fear wasn't about my mortality, it was about my wife's.

Her

Elke had suggested during our first visit that I might have post-traumatic stress as a result of my cancer, and that what I was experiencing was anxiety, but I didn't hear her with my true self. The last session was when I truly grasped that what I was experiencing was anxiety. My eyes teared up and it all just came together. It made sense now.

Each time I saw Elke, I understood what she was saying and tried each new tool, but I wasn't really seeing it. I finally had a great understanding of what was happening when I created an imaginary locked box for my worries. Even now, I can't say that "my worries" stay there, live there or will even always be there, but that's where I put them for now. That's where they'll be if I need them.

Which moment changed me? To be frank, all of them. From crying about my cancer with a lavender tissue dabbing my nose, the sound of a singing bowl healing my thoughts, to even using eye movement desensitization and reprocessing. Each visit I gathered as many tools as Elke would teach me, and envisioned them as life skills. She is elite and full of wisdom and experience and grace. She is Elke. I still to this day refer to her as my life coach, however, she truly is our Anxiety Warrior.

Amanda shares more about her pre-treatment journey through the medical care system in "I'll Be Fine" (page 224) in this book.

When Anxiety Encounters Traditional Chinese Medicine

Kory Sadie Ford

On a daily basis, I meet and treat people suffering from a wide variety of health issues. Patients come to me to discuss everything from acne to infertility, in various stages of life from infancy into their elder years.

I practice as a registered Traditional Chinese Medicine Practitioner, in Guelph, Ontario. Traditional Chinese Medicine (TCM) has many different tools, from acupuncture to dietary/herbal therapy, as well as cupping, *Tui Ni* (massage), and other muscular-skeletal treatment modalities. I have yet to meet a clinical condition that TCM can't help, and so many other conditions that are not yet serious enough to be considered as western clinical conditions, but which are wreaking havoc in people's lives. There are also those who come to see me because "something is just not right."

The power of TCM lies in its ability to differentiate between conditions. As we now know, anxiety can look and feel like a lot of different things. It has a spectrum. In general the condition, in the view of TCM, has an affect on the Shen, which can be defined loosely as our spirit and our general sense of vitality. The Shen is stored and governed by the heart.

There are many different approaches to addressing any condition in TCM. For the purpose of this conversation, I'll simplify things by looking at anxiety only through the elemental system, developed by J.R. Worsley.[1]

Worsley's approach is based on observations by the ancients that the fundamental elements of creation—wood, fire, earth, metal, and water—create life's natural, mysterious order. When these five elements within us are in a balanced and harmonious state, wrote Worsley, we experience health, well-being and the joy of being alive.

According to his teachings, the cause of our physical, mental, and spiritual distress resides within us rather than in external circumstances.

These elements are associated with organs in our body as well as emotional states. Anxiety primarily affects the following organs:

✦ Spleen: Earth—excessive worry and rumination.

✦ Liver: Wood—frustration.

✦ Kidney: Water—fear.

✦ Heart: Fire—anger.

✦ Lung: Metal— grief and the inability to let go.

Sometimes anxiety will come about simply because one of the organ systems becomes out of balance. However, in this five-element approach all of us have a constitutional/causative factor (CF). Our CF is with us from birth to death. It is our coloured lens through which we view the world. One could compare it to our astrological sign, or the results of a Myers-Briggs assessment, or any other personality-based assessment of how we approach situations and make our way through the world. This gives us an idea or understanding of why different patterns of anxiety exist. (To find out your CF, visit my website www.eastmeetswesthealth.ca, located under the "Resources" tab.)

Here are two examples: one pattern of anxiety stems from:

✦ Kidney "qi" deficiency. The energy of the kidneys is too low. This pattern of anxiety will manifest as preoccupation and feelings of fear or dread. It can be accompanied by lower back and knee weakness and a lack of sexual responsiveness.

✦ Lack of strength in the lungs manifests as rapidly changing moods, an inability to let go, aversion to speaking, shortness of breath, fatigue, and sweating easily upon exertion.

My first experience with full-blown anxiety came on a beautiful July day. I was in my early 20s and on my way to work. The previous year I had completed an Honours Bachelor of Science degree at the

University of Guelph and set out to find work within the scientific community. I passed over several jobs with great wages and benefits, as they were within the scientific community but focused on sales. Having decided that participating in actual science was more important to me than having a high-paying job, I took a position in a biochemical laboratory that analyzed samples for veterinary clinics.

On that particular July day when my anxiety began, I had come to the realization that I would never move up in the company and that I had learned as much as I could in my position. I am a wood/earth CF, and people of this type are soothed by goal setting and moving forward in life. Like a healthy tree, the roots grow deep into the earth, meandering around rocks (obstacles).

Traffic came to a grinding halt, which was the straw that broke the camels back. The combination of not moving forward literally and in the bigger scheme of life brought on a massive panic attack. I could not get enough air, I had a gripping pain in my chest, and my body started to shake. I pulled off the road and had a talk with myself; that day I submitted my notice.

Quitting or abandoning a project is not always possible or the right decision. I could have kept the job and found another aspect of my life to express my need for growth. One thing I have learned from Chinese medicine above all else is moderation. If we are constantly moving and growing, the wood energy will become exhausted. North American culture, at least at this point, will rarely pat you on the back for taking a day for yourself or for coming in second place.

If we really want to achieve good mental, physical, and emotional health, we need to be our own "gold star" providers; our own back patters.

We need to find contentment in stillness. I did not understand this until some time in my 30s, when my wood energy was totally depleted from completing many programs and specializations while working multiple jobs to support all of my goals. This was when I came to understand the earth aspect of my constitution. A dirty combination, I might add. The wood is busy making all kinds of plans for the earth element to continually ruminate about. Earth types are care providers by nature (this explains most of my poor relationship choices). An out-of-balance earth type will put all others' needs ahead of their own.

Finding a partner who wanted me rather than needed me was a key part in addressing my anxiety. Creating a safe space for me to draw my personal boundary lines, and taking part in healthy activities in which I could be a helper (volunteering and clinical work), and feeling heard have also become important tools that aid in my system re-balancing. Fostering strong and open communication within my relationships is a lifelong goal.

This brings me to mantras, for me the best and most powerful way to use my voice. For you it may be church choir, rocking out in the car, or screaming at the top of your lungs at a rock concert. The earliest mantras were composed in Vedic Sanskrit by the Hindus of India over 3000 years ago[2]. Mantras are melodic phrases with spiritual interpretations that have psychological or spiritual powers to alter our states of mind. I have had amazing experiences both personally and in group settings reciting a mantra. The language often still feels very foreign to me, but the emotional release that I have seen and the physiological changes in my body have far surpassed most other measures I have taken to address my anxiety and overall health.

Food is another powerful tool we all can use every day to balance energies in the body. Food is medicine. One of the side effects of being an earth CF is that when out of balance, we can tend to obesity. Looking back, I have come to realize that an operation I had at age five and subsequent steroidal medications were the beginning of my earth energy coming out of balance. By 12 years of age I was 79 kg (about 175 lbs), which of course brought on anxiety surrounding body image. From then until my late 20s, when I started studying Chinese medicine, I tried every western medical approach to weight loss. None seemed effective for me, and this proved particularly frustrating as I was working as a personal training and fitness instructor.

Chinese medicine illustrated to me that I needed to view food in a totally different way: it needed to become a part of me. My focus switched from weight loss to nourishment. If I was too hot, I ate cooling foods; if deficient in energy, I ate foods to build strength. Not only did I pay attention to the types of foods I was ingesting, but also to the way in which I was preparing them and my mental state during preparation.

I was able, through diet therapy, to build the strength of my digestive system so that I was finally able to absorb the nourishment from the food I was putting in my mouth. Since then, I have not stepped on a scale unless I found myself becoming too thin. My weight, although it still fluctuates, will not likely ever be a concern for me again. Food is no longer an enemy, but a kind, warm, and nourishing ally. Also, depending on the anxiety pattern that you have, even a small amount of a particular food can exacerbated your internal pattern, so it's best to approach most foods in moderation, and a few of them not at all.

Finally, the last piece to my anxiety puzzle was to find movement that worked for me. In TCM when there is *Qi* or blood deficiency—a common characteristic in the wood element—energy may stagnate in the body. Therefore, movement is essential. However, too much or too aggressive forms of exercise will consume more *Qi* and blood, causing more stagnation. Moderation is the key.

My advice to anyone would be to find the type of movement that makes you happy in your heart. When we connect with our Shen, movement becomes effortless. It is the form of movement that will make an hour pass in what seems like five minutes. Depending on my available energy, bodyweight workouts, walking and free style dance are my correct formula. The next time you are exercising and catch yourself smiling with your eyes and your heart, you will know you have found a good form of movement for you.

In conclusion, it is first important to know and learn about who we are in the world, what drives us, what we like and dislike. What non-ideal patterns do we seem to repeat *ad nauseam*, despite them not aiding us in our life journeys? Once we have some idea of where we we are coming from, we can find our tools:

✦ Appropriate movement (yoga, walking, dance).

✦ Foods that feel good to ingest, and make us feel good after ingesting (e.g., raw vs. cooked, thermal properties, flavours).

✦ A form of emotional release (mantra).

Once we are given a western diagnostic label such as anxiety, we often feel it is a permanent, lifelong assignment. TCM shows us that disease has a spectrum, so although the pattern behind our anxiety may always on some level be present, our tools can keep the system balanced, so to not let the anxiety manifest.

Notes

1   J.R. Worsley (2000), The Five Elements and the Officials, Red Wing Book Company, Ed. 2.
2   Jan Gonda (1963), The Indian Mantra, Oriens, Vol. 16, pages 244-297.

The Masks We Wear

Karen Girard

I got the weirdest phone call... It was the receptionist from a walk-in clinic I had been to a couple of weeks earlier. She said, "Your results have been confirmed." But more on that later.

Anxiety raises its ugly head in many ways. It is not just the crippling panic attacks, or the veil that comes down over your thoughts, or making you forget everything you know in an exam. It is not just the heart palpitations, sweats, trouble breathing, or being unable or unwilling to go out in a crowd.

Anxiety can also mean assuming a mask—hiding your true being, not wanting to be seen for who you are because you feel you are not good enough and that you are always being judged. Think about teenagers trying so hard to fit in that they do things they know they shouldn't.

This has been my life.

Many would call me an extrovert, speaking to everyone I meet. True, it is one of my characteristics, but truth be told, I am a pleaser—always trying to fit in and be liked, often nattering about nothing in particular just to look like I belong somewhere.

Anxiety is a cruel master that can rob you of your very identity.

My teens: a funny-looking kid with glasses and braces (head-gear!). I was bullied and didn't easily make friends at school. I wasn't smart enough for the smart group, or cool enough for the cool group. The cheerleaders didn't let me join them because I wasn't allowed to shave my legs.

I ended up as a member of the "outsiders" group, smoking cigarettes on the hill by the school and using recreational drugs. This group didn't care much about me, as long as I had money and smokes to share. The mask I put on was tough, uncaring about what others thought about me, and completely opposite to who I really was. It was better than being alone though, or so I thought.

Early adulthood: 28 years ago, when I married my husband, he suggested that I stay home with the children.

I realize this would be a dream come true for many. But for me? I had worked my whole life and my identity at that time was tied to my career. Did I tell him that? No, I put on the mask of being the perfect mom and wife, meeting everyone else's expectations at the expense of my own. Don't get me wrong. I loved having time to spend with my babies and watching them grow into smart, funny people, but inside I envied my husband. We had met at college, and he now had the career that we both had trained for.

Twelve years later, I was a stay-at-home mom with all my children in school. While I was volunteering, I often spent many of my days at home alone.

When I broached going back to work part-time, my husband said, "But we agreed you would stay home."

My response: "No, you agreed, and I just went along with it because I thought if I didn't, you would love me less."

This was my first step out from behind a life-long mask created by my social anxiety as a child.

In 2011, as my children were becoming young adults and beginning to fly the coop, I realized that I had totally lost sight of "me." Like many women at this stage, I had invested all my time and energy into my beautiful family. I have no regrets there, but now the children didn't need me as much, and that left me with a lot of time on my hands. I didn't know what I liked to do anymore, and I felt very lost. I reverted to earlier bad habits of smoking (and hiding it like a teenager), watching junk TV, and avoiding going out of the house.

Socially, I felt I had nothing to add to a conversation. My anxiety led me to poor health and dark places. Anti-depressants seemed to help the mood a bit, but I needed something to get me out the door and into life.

After an accident that left me alone at home, foot in the air, unable to walk, Facebook and video games got me through the day. This was my social contact—anonymous "creeping" around what everyone else (who, I felt, had the life I wanted) was doing. I was an early adopter of online socialization and lived my social life through screentime. If only I could make myself take that step outside.

At that time, telesummits were becoming popular, and while I was still laid up I tuned in to "Women On Purpose" and listened to Janet Bray Attwood talking about the Passion Test.

The Passion Test is a tool that helps people identify their top five passions—the things that are most important to have as a part of their life, so they can learn where to focus their time and live a more fulfilling life. Sounds perfect, doesn't it? I didn't know what I liked, and I needed someone to help me get there.

It was then that I realized I had to take a step out of my comfort zone, beyond my social mask, and learn about me.

Not one to think before I act, I took a leap of faith and signed up for the Passion Test Facilitator Program almost 2000 km away in Los Angeles. Never mind that I had not even experienced the test myself, I just knew that it was something that I wanted to be a part of. Not only did I not have the money for it, but I also had to get there, share a room, and be vulnerable in a group of complete strangers. As soon as I hit Pay Now, the real anxiety appeared.

What would my husband say? I didn't even consider him when I was taking money from the family account for something I had heard about online, let alone planning a trip alone, away from the kids... and assuming that he would be fine with taking care of them on his own. Who else would be there? I bet they were all experienced speakers, with great lives. Would anyone like me?

My husband is very generous, and I know he wouldn't have said no had I asked, but once again I was afraid. I told him in a very offhand way, when we were out for dinner with friends.

Actually, I told my friend, and just assumed that he had heard (I said that out loud, right?)... but that is a story for another time.

The Passion Test weekend was my first step at reclaiming my identity and my life. My number one passion coming out of the event was to "Courageously be true to myself and what I want, without worrying about what anyone else thinks." No more walking on eggshells. Having gone through the process, putting it down on paper, and affirming it to the group was the first step in lifting my veil and living my truth.

Anxiety is often brought on by false ideas, false beliefs and false concepts—the same things that prevent us from living a passionate life. Our emotions and feelings are there to protect and guide us. I discovered that my anxiety was really a tool I used as self-protection. What I went on to learn was that there were other, better tools to help me manage my anxiety.

Anxiety isn't a completely bad thing. It is usually caused by a fear of the unknown, and what we believe could or may happen. With traffic lights, the red light is meant to keep us safe. When it comes to anxiety, the "red light" appears prematurely. We need to determine whether a red light (stop everything!) is really required.

I learned to consider the first appearance of my anxiety symptoms as a yellow light—an indication to pause or slow down, and proceed with caution. Easier said than done, right? This is where other tools come in. (For more on these tools, see "What I Learned from the Passion Test" at the end of this chapter.)

The Passion Test

The Passion Test was the beginning of a huge life change for me. My experience with it was so positive that I wanted to share it not only with other adults, but also with the youth I worked with in the school system. Wouldn't it be amazing if they could begin to learn these things and use them as part of their lives? I went on to become a Level 1 Master Trainer for the Passion Test for Kids and Teens, and began to deliver workshops in leadership classes and conferences in addition to the adult Vision Board and Passion Test workshops I started with.

In October 2013, I took my next huge leap and did a TedX talk: "Using Passion to Inspire Action in Education." While on stage, I mentioned that I had never taken art classes as I didn't have the time.

Be careful what you send out to the universe.

In November 2013, I found a lump in my chest. Three months earlier, a mammogram and ultrasound had detected nothing. When I spoke with a doctor about it, she believed it was just another cyst. I have fibrocystic breast disease, so lumps are common.

Every night I would fiddle with this lump, feel it growing and try not to worry, but while controlling my anxiety I was not listening to my intuition or advocating for myself. I believed a doctor knows best, so that I shouldn't second guess. I should have asked for another opinion or a test.

I went to a doctor again in February, and was reassured again that all was likely fine, as my mammogram had been clear in August. In March, I went to a walk-in clinic.

Fast forward to Holy Thursday 2014, the day before Good Friday and the Easter long weekend. I got the weirdest phone call. It was the receptionist from the walk-in clinic. She said, "Your results have been confirmed."

"So it is just a fibroadenoma?"

"No (pause), it's breast cancer."

"Oh. Does it say anything about what stage or anything?"

"It says something about III/III."

"I don't know what that means. What should I be doing?"

(Pause) "Um, maybe you should speak to the doctor..."

Duh!!! Okay, how was she to know that no doctor had been in touch with me?

I was new to this, so I didn't know how most people learned about diagnoses like this, but I am pretty sure it isn't dropped like a bomb the day before every place is closed for the long weekend so you can't learn more until after Easter Monday. Talk about anxiety inducing!

Two years earlier, before the Passion Test, I would have been paralyzed with fear.

Instead, I took deep breaths and considered what could happen. Yes, the worst, but also the other options. Without seeing the doctor, I could not determine how likely these things were, but I knew that my map of reality would guide me along the way.

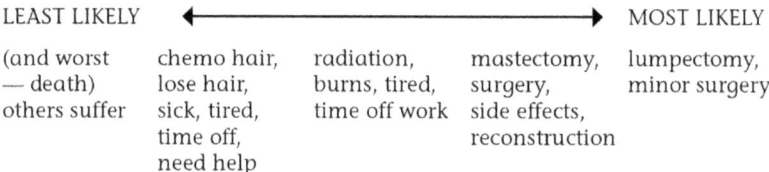

LEAST LIKELY	←————————————————————→			MOST LIKELY
(and worst — death) others suffer	chemo hair, lose hair, sick, tired, time off, need help	radiation, burns, tired, time off work	mastectomy, surgery, side effects, reconstruction	lumpectomy, minor surgery

My map of reality with cancer was not good. I had helped take care of my father when he was dying from skin cancer. A month before, his sister had died from breast cancer. It was terrifying to think about. On the other hand, my mother was a survivor, and I knew others who were, too.

I also knew my children were watching me, and I wanted to show them that you can go through adversity with grace and courage. I needed to be a role model.

On went another mask, one of courage and self-sufficiency. Even though I did not feel that confident, I believe this mask helped me as much as it helped my children. It was a more positive one.

I believe that the work I had been doing for the past two years, using the Passion Test and learning to manage my anxiety, actually saved my life.

Instead of panicking and going inside myself to those dark places, I began to look for other tools that would help guide me.

A couple of days earlier, I had put aside a piece of mail that looked interesting. It turned out to be a brochure for an organization called

Wellspring. Wellspring is a network of support centres offering programs and services that meet the emotional, social, practical, and restorative needs of people living with cancer and those who care for them. These programs are offered free of charge.

The brochure was sitting beside my chair as I was writing my list of what could happen. While taking a break, I was drawn to the brochure, read it, and learned about services that were available to support cancer patients and their families.

Next to the diagnosis, visiting Wellspring was probably one of the most anxiety-ridden things I had done in a long time. I knew what was coming—surgery and chemotherapy—but somehow making the trip to the Wellspring house and crossing that threshold felt like an admission: I have cancer.

The mask that I had been wearing for my family was also covering up my real fears.

Admitting I needed support was another major tool in dealing with my anxiety. As I walked through Wellspring's door, my eyes welled with tears, my stomach seemed to jump to my throat, and I really wanted to turn and run. Instead, I went in and asked for the help I needed.

Sometimes, we do fine using the tools we have to manage anxiety. Other times, we have to admit that we need more help. Help is out there, if only you look for and ask for it. People cannot support you unless you let them know that you need it.

Wellspring became "my place," full of people going through the same thing as me, and workers who understood what we patients were going through, and were able to support us. It was at Wellspring that my next passion was nurtured.

Remember when I put out to the universe that I had never had time to do art? Wellspring had some amazing art programs, all for free. I had never done art, and now not only did I have time, but I also had teachers, materials, a studio—everything I needed to get started.

Strange. Cancer actually held a gift—time to pursue art. I have since taken up intuitive art, and while not being an "artist," have sold a couple of my paintings, have them showing in a coffee house, and sell cards and other items with my artwork on it.

Best of all, I took off the mask of victim, and began following my passions. Discovering colour was just the beginning. On the verge of retirement, I took a step out and went back to school for expressive arts training through the Prairie Institute of Expressive Art Therapy.

My mask is off and I am following my passions. I am alive, and doing what I can with the life that I have. Am I afraid of what may come next, of recurrence? Absolutely, and then I bring myself back to the present, look around me, and see the gifts...

... and if I need a change, I pull out my paints, get my hands dirty, and finger paint my feelings onto a canvas.

What I learned from the Passion Test

One of the tools I learned through the Passion Test was to understand and regulate my anxiety using "Nature's Guidance System." Listening to your body is a chance to take control by being aware of the contraction and expansion in your life. Anyone can do this. Give it a try.

The first step is to notice. What are your signs that anxiety is coming on? Do you get heart palpitations, feel overheated, sweat, and have brain fog, tension in your jaw or neck, or back pain? Is it the voice inside your head that gets louder than reality? When we pay attention to our own bodies and know our signs, we can begin to notice and acknowledge these before a full-on attack has a chance to come on.

Next, start managing your breath. Breathe. When we are anxious we often either begin taking shallow breaths and don't get enough oxygen to the brain, or breathe too deeply and fast, and get too much (yes, there really is such a thing, which is why you see people breathing into a bag). When you have this shortness of breath, you are actually hyper oxygenated. Your body can't absorb all the oxygen. It's like hyperventilating. By slowing your exhalation, your body has time to replace the oxygen with CO_2. There always has to be a balance of both in your body.

When a friend saw me having an anxiety attack, she gave me this specific exercise: Take a large breath in and exhale as slowly as possible, counting to 25. Do this at least six times. Repeat as needed. As you practice you should be able to do it longer. If you are struggling with anxiety-related shortness of breath, this may be hard to do at first. With anxiety-related shortness of breath, you constantly feel the urge to yawn. Yawning slows your breathing and gives you relief. Now that you are breathing a bit better, ask yourself to be open to possibilities, and not just to the "voice" in your head.

Let yourself feel the feelings.

Anxiety is worsened by pushing feelings away, avoiding or being frightened by them. It is okay to let yourself feel them, and as you do,

✦ Ask yourself: "What is the worst that could happen?" and write it down.

✦ Ask again, "What else could happen?"

✦ Do this a few times, then write the answers along a scale based on how likely each is to happen. This may make it more realistic for you.

LEAST LIKELY ←————————————————→ MOST LIKELY

✦ Next, ask yourself what is the worst that could happen for each of the situations on your scale... and then what, and then what.

As you think through the scenarios, you may find that the worst may not be all that bad, and you can prepare for it with an action plan.

Use the tools you already rely on to manage anxiety. As this process becomes more automatic, you will develop a better sense of what works best for you. Make up a list of some of the specific tools that work for you, and start making changes. Categories and examples of tools include:

✦ Physical: Exercise, go for a walk outside, dance, do breathing exercises.

✦ Mental: Meditate, pray.

✦ Emotional: Talk to somebody, cry, let it out, cuddle your puppy.

✦ Spiritual: Meditate, pray, draw, write, anything that works for you.

Please refer to Support Chart (page 294) to use this approach.

House of Cards to Happiness

Tracey Howarth

When I used to think about anxiety, I would think of panic attacks, obsessive compulsive tendencies, or agitation. I surfed through my early adult life feeling unsettled, frustrated, easily angered, unhappy, and unsatisfied. But I never thought I had anxiety. I became to believe this was just my personality.

At age 19, I attended college to become a paramedic. It was never a career that I had dreamt of pursuing, but with my background as a lifeguard, taking a one-year program to become a paramedic seemed like an easy choice.

I remember being at college and wondering about the program choice I had made. Was this a career path that I was truly meant to be in? Did this career choice fuel my soul? Was it something I could actually do for the next 30 years? I remember my dad telling me, "Tracey, it doesn't matter if you ever work as a paramedic, but it is important to finish the program." So, I did. I graduated with honours on the Dean's list and passed my provincial exam. The next logical step was finding work, as I didn't know what I wanted to do next. I was hired at the local ambulance service in my small town, and there I stayed for almost 18 years.

I remember the first summer, feeling terror every time I was dispatched on a call. I remember knowing that being a paramedic was not my calling, and trying to figure out what I could do instead. But before I knew it I had purchased a house and got married. And in another blink of an eye I had a toddler, a farm, and I was well into my 30s. This was the height of my anxiety. My job terrified me, my toddler overwhelmed me, and my marriage was crumbling.

Every day I was angry, overwhelmed, irritable. I struggled to find happiness. Negativity and intolerance were my persona. I remember my boss giving me a gag gift one day, a pink polka dot magnet that said, "My greatest fear is there is no PMS and this is my personality."

At the time I thought it was funny and fitting. In retrospect it was sad, and should have been a wake-up for me. I was on a sad spiral of unhappiness, and I had absolutely no idea how to stop it or change it. So instead I buried it. I blamed my husband, snapped at my toddler, and counted down my days until my next day off, to my next holidays, and to my retirement.

Only a couple years after I started working, my father was killed in an accident. On the advice of my doctor, I started taking anti-anxiety and depression medications to help me with my unbearable grief. I still didn't "feel" like I had anxiety. I am not even sure that I knew at that time what anxiety felt like. I was sad, and I kept telling myself that the tingling, heart-racing I felt at work was adrenalin, and since I had chosen the field of paramedicine I was clearly an adrenalin junkie. This is part of the uniform.

My heart would drop when the pager went off. I would will myself to take secret deep breaths on the way to calls. I would struggle to remain composed in difficult situations. I would spend my days off sleeping, and would dread waking up to my alarm, when it was still dark outside, driving to work in the dark, and driving home in the dark.

As time marched on I still could not shake the feeling I had had when I was in college. I felt unsettled, dissatisfied, and unhappy. I had no reason to. I had a wonderful life. I had a beautiful farm, husband, an incredible daughter, and a lovable Labrador retriever.

I retreated to the barn to hide from life. I began training to show my horses and it took all my free time and money. Being in the barn with my horses was the only time I felt alive. I avoided my marital problems and spent time with the horses instead. The barn fed my soul. Galloping on the back of a half-tonne (1,000 lb.) animal gave me a different adrenalin rush, one that felt right, one that felt like me.

At work, I was good at my job. I was a great paramedic. I had a partner who made me laugh, and had my back at all times. I had coworkers that I could trust and knew would be there if we needed them. I was paid well and had a lot of vacation time. But deep down inside, I was afraid to admit I hated my job.

My job continued to terrify me. I still had heart palpations every time the pager went off. I would break out in sweat halfway through my shift. I sometimes shook and had to take deep breaths on the way to calls. But once on the call, I was confident, calm and capable. I was the paramedic you wanted. I was a fierce patient advocate, and extremely empathic.

When I returned from a difficult call, I pretended that I was okay. I laughed off horrible things I'd seen. I would say, "It's fine."

I've seen things that cannot be unseen, and heard things that cannot be unheard. I vowed to myself to never bring my work home. The moment I got in my car at the end of shift, I had the drive home to decompress, and that was it. When I walked into the house, I would be me, not Paramedic me. I never talked about work at home. Legally I am not able to. Privacy laws prohibit me from sharing details about the calls I've done throughout my day.

As I walked into my front door, I would immediately shed my jacket and kick my boots into the back of the closet. I changed out of my uniform as quickly as I could. I told myself I did this because I didn't want to bring work germs into the house. But my inner voice was telling me something different. I was unknowingly carrying around many burdens quietly, and inevitably my marriage was paying the price.

When my husband and I separated, it should have been another wake-up call for me. I spent hours in therapy trying to figure out why my marriage was failing, but never did I look inside myself. My fragmented marriage was a symptom of my anxiety, and still I didn't get it. I was working on "anger issues" and "accepting the separation." Never was it mentioned to me that anxiety and work-related stress were the cause of my marriage issues. If the issue came up in therapy, I would shoot it down.

"I'm good at my job, it can't be that."

"Get out! Get out! It's making you sick," my inner voice would scream.

"Impossible! I need this job, it pays too well."

This inner monologue went on for years.

With a lot of work, my husband and I were able to reconcile and move forward in a much healthier marriage. I suppose I subconsciously was 'getting it.'

I became happier in my marriage, but still felt unsatisfied in life.

The universe was unhappy with me. I was stifling my inner voices, so I had one last loud wake-up call on a sunny morning in May. It forever changed my life's path.

While on my way home from a night shift, still in uniform, I happened upon a horrific motorcycle incident, and quickly realized the injured person was someone I knew. Despite my best efforts, I knew this person would die from their injuries. I went home numb, and my shell cracked open.

As a result of the incident, I suffered crippling anxiety and was diagnosed with PTSD. I was unable to return to work as a paramedic.

I had been living in a delicate house of cards for many, many years. That sunny morning my house came crashing down, and I had to take a good hard look at my life and figure out what to do next. My inner voice was screaming at me, anxiety symptoms took control of my body, and I could not ignore them any longer.

I experienced flashbacks, a racing heart, sudden uncontrolled shaking. I suffered through surprise crying fits, and hypervigilance. Driving down the highway caused me distress. (What if there was an accident, would I stop? What would I do?) I avoided public pools and beaches, where kids played freely. (What if their parents are not watching them? What if one of them drowns? What would I do?)

I had nightmares and difficultly sleeping. I needed to make a change, and to change now.

Again, I sought therapy and, finally, found someone who understood, very plainly, what was wrong with me. I had been suffering through minor traumas my whole adult life, stuffing away my anxiety. My therapist was unsurprised at my current state. She congratulated me for coping well for so long.

"Tracey, it wasn't a matter of if this would happen, it was a matter of when," she told me in our first session. It was then, I realized, I needed to face the demons. And face them today.

The first six months of therapy were intensive, and focused on decompressing my brain and caring for my physical body. I spent as much time as possible with my horse, I practiced yoga three times a week, and I slept when I was tired, even if it was two o'clock in the afternoon. I was encouraged to do all these things without guilt.

Seven months after I left work, I was feeling physically better. I had decompressed, and most of my symptoms had decreased. However, when I thought about returning to work, I felt panic. *What if I was knocked off the rails again? Could I recover?*

I spent a lot of my therapy sessions tossing around returning to work, or not returning to work. I physically felt great. I was happy and felt settled. I felt the best so far in my adult life. So naturally, I thought it was time to go back to work. Not going back did not seem like an option. What else would I do? What other profession would give me the pay, the time off and the status? If I quit my job, how would that affect my family? What kind of sacrifices would we all have to make? It just didn't feel right to me. I felt the obligation to return to work and return to my full income. But the thought of returning to the job that had slowly broken me was terrifying.

My therapist challenged me to think about not returning to paramedicine. What? Impossible. I remember laughing at the suggestion.

What else would I do? I'm trained to do one thing: care for people in the pre-hospital setting. I had few transferable skills, and few options for modified work. What else would provide me with a steady healthy income, good benefits and a cushy pension? It was impossible to think of anything that would. But she challenged me to think of a different future, following my 'passion.'

"What if you could make your own career by following your passion," my therapist asked.

"It would never pay me enough," I snapped back.

"What if it would? What if you could find a job following your passion, making the same amount of money as before," she challenged.

The next moment is one that I will never forget.

I looked her straight in the eye, and I said, "I don't mean to be offensive, but, following your "passion" isn't for people like me, it's for "arty" people like you."

She laughed wholeheartedly and assured me that the notion is for everyone. And she truly believed I could achieve it. I was the only one holding me back.

I left, and I thought, "This woman has saved me. She has put her heart and soul into rehabilitating me. She has helped me put myself back together. The least I could do is humour her and do what she asked me to do. So I did. I would hold those thoughts, I would figure out my passions, I would toss them out into the universe, and I would come back and prove her wrong; that these notions are not practical for science-based people like me.

I spent a lot of time being aware of what fuelled me. I thought about what I wanted my future to look like (even if it was only a fantasy).

I came up with a list:

+ Work for myself.

+ Stay in health care.

+ Earn decent compensation.

+ Have a dynamic and changing career.

+ Have different options within the career choice.

The bonus list included horses.

I came up with massage therapy, adding equine massage therapy to my skill set. At this point it was still a fantasy. I had no clue how I would ever achieve that goal. The thought was overwhelming. But the more I carried the thought, slowly it did seem achievable. Maybe this was something I could actually do.

I spoke to friends about what I was contemplating, and funny things started to manifest. I heard about people looking for massage therapists. I was offered two jobs if I graduated. My friend and equine chiropractor rejoiced by saying, "We need an equine massage therapist in the area." And almost everyone I spoke to encouraged me to make the change. Be brave, just do it!

So I did.

I went back to college full time at age 37. I quickly found that I was good at it, and I loved it.

During my second semester, I took a four-day course on equine massage therapy. I became a Certified Equine Massage Therapist. I began treating my horses, and my friends' horses, and I loved it. Even better, I was good at it.

Currently, I am still in school and will graduate next year. I am not even a little worried about earning a respectable income. I am so excited about my future. I am the happiest I've been in my adult life. I feel fulfilled, settled, and confident about my future.

My anxiety symptoms have almost completely disappeared. I have the tools to know what to do when a symptom crawls back in. I have goals and an incredibly supportive network of family and friends. Anxiety does not follow me around all day long. I have my triggers, and know when to expect them. I know they will probably be with me for the rest of my life, and that's okay. They are part of me and the journey I've been on.

I know that a future in emergency medicine is no longer for me. Only two percent of paramedics make it to their retirement date. I always thought I would be one of them, but now I know why only two percent make it. I'm okay with it. I am okay with not being in a job where I am counting down the days until retirement. I don't believe that is any way to live.

My hopes are that I have chosen a career path which will allow me to work for as long as I want, and that a pension is not required, in the traditional sense of the word. What if you are able to have a job that you are excited to wake up to every morning? That you don't have to retire from? I am truly happy.

To me, that is the best thing in the world.

Pushing Through My Diagnosis

Meaghan O'Neill

Every day I struggle to understand and deal with my anxiety. This began even before a doctor gave me the diagnosis. I hope that by reading this someone will be able to relate and realize they are not alone. I used to feel isolated from the rest of the world because of my anxiety. I thought that no one else could possibly relate to the racing and sometimes irrational thoughts that were clouding my mind.

As a person with anxiety, I know the daily struggle is real, but it isn't something to be faced alone. I hope that this testimonial brings that feeling to light. You are not alone in your anxiety. You can and will find people who will support you and try to understand your feelings.

I do not have any amazing ideas or revelations when it comes to dealing with anxiety, but I have a story to share. Every day is different. I am not as in control of my anxiety as I wish to be, but I feel that most people struggle with this also.

The anxiety diagnosis devastated me. I thought of myself as an irrational person who could not control her own life. People would avoid me because of what I have since learned to see as an illness. I lived in denial that my anxiety was a problem. I thought, "I'm not anxious; everyone is just pissing me off."

It would start with something small. For example, I am making my lunch for the next day. I drop something, I can't find something else. All of a sudden, I feel overwhelmed with the 5,000 things I need to do before I can go to bed. I start yelling at people and slamming doors because somehow that seems like the best way to handle it.

My head was full of, "You failed, you can't do this right, how stupid can you be?" I became fixated on my own failures, and could not possibly see any of the things I was doing right.

When it finally came to a head, all I could do was cry—at work, at school, at home, with friends, in front of everyone. "There you go again Meaghan, you can't even act like an adult. Can you not see how people are looking at you now?" Which was always followed by intense feelings of guilt and embarrassment. How do you come back from that?

Two of the hardest things for me to overcome were accepting that I had anxiety, and asking for help. Learning to realize when I'm feeling overwhelmed and to take five minutes to bring myself out of the loop of anxious thoughts and feelings. It is difficult in the moment to realize why you are feeling the way you are, and then have the mental awareness to realize what you need to do.

For me, I find that taking my dog for a hike in the bush or sitting in my hammock watching a movie are ways I can calm down after a rough day. In the moment, I can take a second, breathe, and reprioritize. Stepping outside and regrounding myself, even for only five minutes, is always helpful, and I always try to listen when people around me comment that maybe I need a break, because I appear more distracted or frustrated than normal.

The diagnosis of anxiety, while helpful in learning to manage it, comes with an undeniable stigma that sometimes affects my medical care. There's no worse feeling than sitting in your doctor's office attempting to convince them that, although you have anxiety, the symptoms you're experiencing indicate something completely unrelated. That feeling when you see a new doctor reading your chart: they note the anxiety diagnosis, shift their assessment, and no longer pay close attention to your symptoms because 'It's just anxiety.'

I am currently living with some digestive difficulties. At first, doctors were helpful, but once they began to run out of ideas, they fell back on 'anxiety'.

It was not until I pushed further and sought additional opinions that I was able to obtain some sort of meaningful diagnosis. That was eight months ago, and I still don't have all the answers I need to help with my medical issues. I ended up seeking out a naturopath who promptly offered potential treatment options. I am now hopeful about seeing positive changes in the near future. I have also had the help of amazing medical and psychological professionals in learning to cope with and manage my anxiety.

I have been fortunate in that I have surrounded myself with amazing and supportive people. Friends who understand that they need to let me sing through my Toronto traffic anxiety, people who understand when I need a big hug, even when I tell them to go away, or the people who can turn anything into a joke. While a diagnosis of anxiety sometimes makes life harder, without it I would have never learned to manage it, so that I can enjoy and thrive in life.

I Got This:
Unlocking Your Instincts

Nancy Osborne

I was recently asked how other people would describe me: bold, confident, spirited, badass? Well that's how they describe my CV, but people have always described me as happy. "How can you be so happy all the time?" is a question I have faced often. But that's also how I've mostly described myself: happy. Were there times of near unbearable anxiety that led to despair? Oh yes, but somehow I kept learning from these times, moving forward and being happy again.

It is only on reflection that I see how my life might be considered by some as that road less traveled and thus exceptionally challenging. Yet it is those very challenges that have brought me to the amazing place in which I now exist. Interestingly, after dealing with the challenges of my early life, many of the subsequent challenges were ones I sought out and took on willingly.

I was given up at birth and adopted at three months of age. My early years were lived in a home where both serious abuse and love co-existed. I believe this is possible and often the case. I have great memories from my childhood and I have other memories so frightening that I suppressed them for years as a means of self-protection. Then, at the age of 16, my life changed drastically. My mother died and my brother was arrested and committed to an institution.

Serious drug abuse had left my brother a violent paranoid schizophrenic, and he would eventually be charged with a myriad of serious criminal offences, including attempted murder. My father had secretly moved on with another woman before my mother died, finding a new family and gradually leaving what remained of our family behind.

By the time I was 17 years old, I thought of myself as an adult, ready to face the world on my own. So, I did. Anxiety? Of course, but even then, I carried each lesson into the next of life's adventures. Each and every one of my adventures was a different mix of good and bad, love and cruelty.

Despite the challenges, or maybe in spite of the challenges, I had always done exceptionally well at school, consistently on the honour roll and in the top 10 of my grade. I finished secondary school, having completed Grade 12 and opted not to return for Grade 13 despite pressure from teachers and guidance counsellors. I left home that year and lived in a campground until it was closed for the winter. Shortly thereafter, still 17, I joined the regular military. Of interest, years later, while working for UNICEF in Sudan, I learned that Canada had been criticized for allowing child soldiers in the regular forces and it was not until the mid 1980s that the military changed the entry age from 17 to 18 in accordance with international law. I had been a child soldier and had something in common with some of the children I would later serve. But I digress.

It was 1975 and I had seen on the news that the RCMP and a few other progressive police departments were taking their first women as full constables. I had always excelled in academics and somehow knew I needed to develop other more physical and tangible skills. Policing sounded perfect and challenging! Of course, the earliest that anyone could be accepted to the RCMP was at 21 years of age. Hmmm, waiting was not really an option.

The military was also taking women into full policing roles that year, and the age to join any branch of the military was 17. Perfect, I could have four full years of experience before deciding if civilian policing was where I should be. When I completed my testing to join the military, I was given an option to join as an officer and have my education paid for, or to attend the elite Royal Military College. No, I was determined; only policing would do. So, in 1975, I joined the Canadian Forces as a private in the Military Police.

This was the first year that women had ever been accepted into this male-only environment. We were not exactly welcomed with open arms, but I did it all: policing in remote areas pursuing bears, cougars, and drunken soldiers; policing in urban high crime areas and ports of call to foreign sailors; barroom brawls; riots; plain clothes investigations; drill instructor; unarmed combat instructor; weapons instructor for every small arm including grenades and anti tank weaponry; commanding specialized national security investigations and surveillance; officer commanding training... the list goes on.

After 21 years of breaking open that cement ceiling, I retired as a major. Anxiety along the way, oh yes; sexual harassment was present in every facet of life. I experienced what today would be defined as rape; there were the extremes of physical exertion, long hours of constantly proving myself, and no senior women as mentors or advisors. So yes, there were times when anxiety almost overwhelmed me, and I was thankful for the lessons of my childhood and unexpected allies along the way. So, new strategies and tactics were learned, and the overcoming of every obstacle was celebrated.

The lessons from my childhood had given me the confidence and voice to excel at whatever I took on; well, almost. Relationships were the exception. This same period saw a failed marriage, a long string of failed and sometimes seriously abusive relationships, and meeting the love of my life with whom I would spend the next few years testing and subconsciously doing all I could to see if he, too, would leave me. Heap on the anxiety and despair. But I had met him and he didn't leave. This time it took more than the lessons from childhood, and I needed to accept professional counselling to clear my path to a healthy relationship. I did the work and now, some 25 years later, I have a relationship with my husband that is the envy of many.

After retiring from the military, I was recruited by the United Nations as one of the first four women ever to provide security analysis and access negotiations for humanitarian operations. This took me to some of the most dangerous and culturally misogynistic places in the world, including Sudan, South Sudan, Afghanistan, Pakistan, Haiti, and Papua New Guinea, just to name a few. Being the first person into emergencies and war zones: no anxiety there, right? But I remained happy and my appreciation for the life I was living grew exponentially.

Before retiring for the second time, I worked for UNICEF Headquarters in New York as the only woman on a small team of five. We covered everything from policy development to responding to every crisis in the world, whether natural or man-made.

So many adventures and lessons learned along that "road less travelled." During these final six years with the UN, I took the lead to customize and provide security training specifically tailored for women. I provided it to a cumulative audience of more than 700 women across more than 20 countries. I recognized that women wanted a holistic approach to the training, including the psychological and emotional aspects of security that impacted their lives. It was time to start the discussion and share some of the many lessons learned throughout my journey. The demand for the training grew exponentially and the program had to be expanded in proportion.

During my final year with UNICEF, three of my five teammates, including our director, died unexpectedly within months of one another. No replacements would arrive for the next seven months and I would take the place of the director as principal security advisor for UNICEF globally. Almost immediately, we lost friends and colleagues to a targeted attack in Somalia and ended up managing more high-level emergencies around the globe than ever before. Stress and anxiety hit an all-time high for me. I found myself exhausted, but grateful for all the past challenges and lessons learned. That, and the support of some very strong allies, carried me through an almost impossible time.

Then came the time to retire again, concluding 40-plus years of being the first and often only woman in the biggest boy's clubs in the world. I was proud, content, and happy.

You may have guessed by now that retirement really doesn't stick with me. Despite that difficult final year with the UN, I knew that what I had developed for training women was an amazing package; a culmination of lessons from my many journeys down the roads less traveled. How could I just put it all on a shelf and not continue to share what I had learned? I cannot remember a single day in my life when I had not learned something. Yes, the path I chose definitely included some pretty significant amounts of anxiety and stress, but it had also led me to a level of confidence and happiness that few are lucky enough to enjoy. Not share this? Not possible.

The present

Along the way I had developed tactics and strategies that enabled me to overcome the challenges that I, as a woman, had confronted in my personal life and in the workplace. What I have come to realize is that although my journey may have been unique, the challenges I faced along the way were not. There are common threads woven into the fabric for women around the world. After retiring for the second time, I knew that I needed to share my experiences and lessons learned along the way. So, I founded "I Got This"—a series of workshops and presentations—as a vehicle to share my messages, while continuing to learn and pass on the messages of other women; inspiring them to embrace their power, overcome their fears, and step into a confidence that ensures they are safe, heard, respected, and happy. And that makes me happy. I am inspired too; inspired by every woman I talk to. I have learned the value of women the world over. A much untapped resource of support, knowledge, and "I got this" ability. So much can be learned from each other, and by supporting one another we hold the key to changing our own ability to manage those things that threaten us and cause us anxiety.

Strategies and tactics

Having spent so much of my life in male-dominated environments, one of my most important lessons has come from other women. I always thought that I was unique, my fears were unique, my anxiety was unique, and my experiences were unique. None of this was true. I am a woman, and like all women I am both vulnerable and strong.

I have learned how very important it is to share our experiences, as well as our ways of coping, overcoming, and succeeding. I have learned the importance of supporting one another and of being supported. So, I share and I ask. Below I share some tactics that have presented themselves to me along my journey: a simple tactic that allows us to identify when someone does not have our best interests at heart, and another that allows us to use who we are to step into our confidence and power.

The first is something I call my "good guy" filter. In our lives, we all know at least one good man, a man who truly respects women. So, if we encounter someone who, on the surface, is charming with words that sound kind and helpful but our instincts are telling us that something is wrong, we need to listen to those instincts and employ the good-guy filter. When we encounter someone, our ears hear their words but our instincts hear their actions. When the two don't match, our instincts begin to sound alarm bells. However, when those alarms don't support what we are hearing, we often suppress them and act only on what we are hearing with our ears. The "good guy" filter helps us reconcile the two.

Let me explain with an example. Imagine a young woman walking along with her hands full of plastic grocery bags. One bag breaks and the groceries from that bag fall to the ground. Your "good guy" sees her stoop to pick them up. Would he offer to help? Of course he would. If she said "no thank you" he might even offer a second time. "Are you sure? I really don't mind." But if she says no again, he will walk away. He might even feel bad that he could not help but he respects her "no" and will not see it as the start to a negotiation. Unlike someone who would not respect her "no," would help anyway, and say something like "Don't be so silly; learn to accept the kindness of others." None of the words is aggressive or sounds unkind, but they do not match the action; the action of disrespecting her 'no'.

Another tactic that I talk about is "owning your tears." When women are asked, during my workshops, why they love being a woman, one of the most common answers is that they can cry and show emotion. We also say that boys should not be discouraged from crying or showing their emotions. So why is it that when we do cry, we are embarrassed and often try to hide our tears or even ourselves if we can't control the tears? I have always been a crier. When I was a child I was told to stop crying or I would be given a good reason to cry. Of course, that only served to increase my tears so I would hide them or hide myself to avoid whatever that other "reason to cry" might be. Yet I continue to cry; I cry when I am happy, I cry when I am sad, I cry when I am angry, I cry when I am embarrassed, I cry when I am hormonal, I cry at sad movies, I cry at music in touching commercials... and the list goes on. Eventually, I realized that I was not unique. Many women cry as I do. So why should it be something to hide just because we have been told we should?

The worst for me has always been when I cried at work. There I was, in a number of testosterone-driven, male-only environments, and sometimes I would get so frustrated or angry that I would cry. I don't usually cry when I am frightened or even physically hurting, but hurt my feelings and you will see my tears. Naturally, that usually ended with me in the washroom trying to stop crying, and the harder I tried to stop the worse it got. By the time I stopped, my face was blotchy and my eyes were red and swollen. For many women, this is a familiar scenario.

But one day after hearing so many other women's stories, I asked myself why I was ashamed of my tears. It was others who perceived them as a sign of weakness. For me, they were usually a symbol of my anger or hurt feelings. I started to notice the occasional picture of a woman with her chin up, anger in her eyes and tears streaming down her face. The tears only emphasized her anger and determination. Wow, maybe it was time to own my tears.

At UNICEF Headquarters in New York, I worked as part of a very small team. The nature of our work meant that we dealt with life and death situations affecting people around the globe. We needed to get along and work as a team. One of the team members could be a bully. I had seen him bully his way with others many times. On one particular occasion, he began to berate and belittle me in an effort to neutralize my opposing opinion. I was angry at his lack of respect and hurt that he would try this on me, a member of his own team. I could feel my eyes starting to burn and the tears welling up, ready to stream down my face. But instead of trying to stop or hide them or walk away and allow the bullying to succeed, I held my chin up, looked him in the eyes and pointed at my own eyes. "Do you see this? This is a symbol of just how angry I am at this moment. You need to listen respectfully to my point of view. You do not need to change yours, but I *will* be heard." A strange thing happened. He backed down. He was no longer entitled to see me as a hysterical woman, and his bullying actions had not had the desired effect. He listened. I don't recall whether he changed his mind, but I do recall that some tears escaped my eyes but did not escalate to sobs and redness. I had owned my tears.

We cry. It is not a voluntary action but a reaction to a stimulus, as is smiling, laughing, or frowning. Tears belong to us and they work with other forms of expression to show others how we feel. So, try owning your tears and see what happens. You are not alone.

Final words

I believe that some of our anxiety comes from what so many of us have been taught: we are the weaker gender, we cower when we feel pain and we are not capable of achieving lofty goals in life. Anxiety is no less real when based on perceptions rather than reality. But if we can recognize reality over perception, then sometimes that anxiety no longer has a foothold. And in reality, women are naturally strong, are able to endure significant pain, and are incredibly capable.

I stopped doubting this when I met women in the worst possible environments in the world, where rape was being used as a tool of war and they were the targets. I was amazed that these women could support one another and take even the slightest opportunity to laugh with one another. They stood taller and prouder than I have ever stood in my life. Women are strong. Women around the world endure unspeakable pain every day and they go on to care for others around them. Women endure the pain of childbirth and often choose to repeat it. Women can take the pain. Women are capable of so much. They are capable of multitasking and doing for others, more than most can ever imagine doing for themselves. They are capable of greatness but don't limit that greatness to themselves. Rather, they share it freely with the ones they love.

Supporting one another and sharing our experiences is vital in the battle against anxiety. Anxiety is fed by many things and fear is certainly one of them: fear of the unknown, fear of our ability to succeed, and certainly fear of being physically overpowered. My happiness comes now when women are inspired to step into their power, overcome their fears, own their voices and follow their passions.

A Caregiver's Chronicle

M. Secord

Well done! Life has been pretty good. Over the years, opportunities have been taken or passed by, experiences indulged in, good friendships nurtured, kids raised and on their own (or soon on their way). You should be eager for what is approaching... retiring from the demands of work, embarking on the list of things you "could" do, instead of the grind of things you "should" do.

But wait a minute. Something is nagging in the back of your mind. You tried to listen to all the advice, saved whenever possible for the day when working became a choice rather than a necessity. You could have done better at saving, but hey, there is a nest egg that will hopefully carry you through the next stage of life. After all, there is so much yet to indulge in, new journeys to embark on. Can you afford to do it all? For how long? What if life takes an unexpected turn?

I'm sure you know someone over age 65 who requires some type of care. The news is worrying... over 70 percent of individuals 65 and over will require some type of care in their lifetime. The cost of our health care is expected to be staggering. I hear the concerns often: Will this happen to me? Will it wipe out my savings? How much will it cost? Can I afford to live long?

I know too well how life can change in a heartbeat. I've lived through the financial and emotional challenges of caring for my own parents. Now, my passion is to use my personal experience caring for my mother's failing health to help others prepare for these challenges.

I'm one of those Baby Boomers, and my story is becoming more common. Our financial anxiety is certainly justified. My own experience leads me to wonder how well this would play out for myself, or most others.

My parents were enjoying retirement together, a busy social life, travel, community work, and a passion for sailing. They were often referred to among their friends as a "power couple." Family visits were complicated to arrange around their hectic schedules, but I felt blessed that they were healthy, independent, and truly happy. In a flash everything changed.

Just seven years ago, I learned of my father's terminal lung disease. He knew more than he was willing to share. His greatest fear was the fate of his 79-year-old wife of 55 years (my mother), who was behaving oddly, showing obvious signs of Alzheimer's disease. There were subtle changes in her behaviour, such as a reluctance to shower, difficulty preparing a meal, and losing her way to places she frequented.

In hindsight, I recalled her calling me several times a day, forgetting that we had just spoken. It wasn't until I visited, and to my complete shock, my mother, who was an outstanding cook, announced dinner was served. Dinner for three consisted of a plate with two fried eggs. I was horrified and realized life as my parents and I knew it was spiraling out of control. I had two young children, a failing marriage, and lived a two-hour drive away. I had no idea how I was going to cope with so much anxiety.

Within five months, I was dealing with my mother's diagnosis of Alzheimer's and my father's sudden passing. I couldn't concentrate on my job, was on medication for anxiety, overwhelmed with grief, all while trying to figure a way out of an abusive relationship. I knew very little about Alzheimer's disease or the journey I was about to embark on.

I didn't feel comfortable knowing my mother was home alone. She lost her independence and mobility when I took her car away. She used telephone banking to pay the same utility bills repeatedly, discarded important documents, and almost set the house on fire defrosting frozen cookies for 45 minutes in the microwave. I sold her car, but she wandered the neighbourhood searching for this only means of independence. I had to arrange for a neighbour to repeatedly run over to hang up the phone that she never remembered to put back in the cradle. Having disconnected the stove and microwave, I arranged for Meals-on-Wheels but she couldn't remember to eat. I was overwhelmed with worry.

As for my mother, she was frustrated with the constant assessments and I had to trick her into attending medical appointments. To complicate matters, my mother was a former registered nurse and college professor, and had acquired a Bachelors Degree in Nursing and a Masters in Education. She possessed the ability to perform many of the tasks during her assessments by mentally preparing her concentration. Combine this with her affable personality, and she was almost able to disguise the severity of her condition.

I had already spent much time managing her care when I should have been earning a living. Within eight months of her diagnosis, I was able to convince my mother to move into a retirement home, where she flourished... for a while. This period provided me the time and energy to end an abusive marriage and focus on the well-being of myself and my children.

This brief respite quickly vanished. My mother was diagnosed with Transient Ischemic Attacks (TIAs), mini-strokes, and soon after, Parkinson's disease. Every week resulted in a "new normal."

My sister and I struggled to keep up with my mother's steady decline and constant changes in her care. Knowing that my mother was safe and supervised had been a great relief, but her physical and mental decline were taking a toll, financially, physically, and emotionally. I fought relentlessly for maximum support from the health care system—a measly one hour a day. I hired a part-time caregiver through an agency, but this new sense of relief lasted only a few months. My mother became less mobile, and safety became more of a priority than companionship.

Assisted living requires its residents to be fairly independent, but my mother could no longer dress herself, collect her medication, or answer the phone. She had no sense of time to attend meals, could not toilet herself or handle her own hygiene, and required prompting to put a forkful of food to her mouth. The amount of money it took to maintain her care was concerning. Paying for a caregiver through an agency was becoming too expensive, so by networking with other residents' families, I was able to hire a full-time private caregiver.

Within four years, my mother had eroded a good chunk of her savings on the cost of her care. Would she outlive her savings? I was concerned about the cost of care but determined to refrain from admitting my mother to a long-term care facility for as long as possible, at least until she was not aware that she was in such a facility. After all, there were times of lucidity, where her own medical background would make her aware of her hopeless situation. I was trying to delay bearing the guilt of such a decision for as long as possible. I started to focus on cost containment so my sister and I alternated caregiving on weekends, but this was taking a physical and emotional toll on us.

We began visiting long-term care facilities, preparing for the inevitable. We researched facilities, learned the system, and spent countless hours learning every detail of care that would be provided during her declining health. The wait list was a shock... three years. How would we cope this long? The ongoing cost of her care would surely be a challenge. More stress, more anxiety.

The day arrived, in 2014, when a bed came available in a facility of our liking. We did what I called the "Dairy Queen run." At least that's where my mother thought she was going. I was relieved when she settled into her new surroundings with little awareness of the change. She was safe and content, so I oddly felt little guilt. With government subsidized care, out-of-pocket costs decreased dramatically.

She continues to exist in the same facility. However, she has no recognition of those she loves, can no longer walk or talk or feed herself, and just recently is challenged with swallowing. I have spent the last few years grieving. I have lost every aspect of my mother except her physical existence. Although each visit is a sad reminder of how much I miss her, I'm convinced she's comforted, on some level, by my presence. Her spirit, intellect, humour, and conversation are all gone, but when our eyes meet I know we're connecting on some level.

This journey could happen to any of us. Not everyone has someone to advocate on our behalf for a decent level of care. Our health care system is bracing for an onslaught of chronic and progressive diseases that will beset the baby boomer generation. Wait times for assisted living and facility care are already staggering. Facilities are regulated, but horror stories of abuse and poor care are shocking. In Ontario, public long-term care facilities are generously subsidized. This won't last long.

This is my personal story. Most of us prefer to live in our own homes as long as possible. I urge everyone to prepare for our later years of poor health. The good news may be that we're living longer, the downside is that our later years may be lived out in poor health.

My mother needed increasing care for several years. Fortunately, she had the financial means to afford what she deserved. Fortunately, she was able to stay in her own home longer than many in her situation. Most of us will not.

Managing my anxiety in a difficult time

This was a period of extreme anxiety for me. I frequently look back and wonder how I coped. My anxiety was mostly attributed to my ability to work and earn an income despite regular interruptions arranging care for my mother. I constantly worried about my mother's situation. My two children, then a preteen and a teenager, also needed my presence and attention, and I tried my best not to neglect their needs.

I drove six hours alternate weekends to care for my mother, often in poor weather. There was little time for self-care, so my sleep, eating, and exercise habits were poor. This led me to worry that I was compromising my own health and well-being. The stress was overwhelming and exhausting.

Here are some of the coping strategies that helped me through this period:

✦ Forcing myself to dedicate a bit of time to doing something that brings comfort and pleasure. (I cherished time late at night, losing myself in magazines and movies.)

✦ Having someone to confide in. It's important to have someone to turn to before the anxiety becomes overwhelming. It can bring a different perspective to the situation that can make coping easier. Fortunately my sister is also a "night owl" and we would spend hours talking on the phone, supporting each other through this journey. If no one can fulfill this role for you, don't hesitate to seek counselling.

✦ Maintaining a "self-care" routine—getting proper sleep, eating right, and going for a walk as often as possible. Don't minimize the importance of these good habits. We can be of little help to others if we are not in good health ourselves.

✦ Accepting help whenever offered and not hesitating to reach out for help on occasion. I occasionally arranged for my mother's caregiver to work an extra day on a weekend to give me a break. It was well worth the extra cost.

+ Humour. Sounds funny, but I had to find some humour in the situation. My mother is light-hearted and possessed a delightful sense of humour. I know she would understand the need to indulge in a good laugh now and then. Occasional comic relief calmed my anxiety and made light of a difficult situation.

+ Networking with others in the same situation. Sharing coping strategies.

+ Seeking out information. For example, not-for-profit organizations such as the Canadian Cancer Society, Parkinson Canada, and Alzheimer Society Canada are great sources of information that can help you understand and plan for your journey.

Financial strategies as we age

There are steps you can take to minimize or prevent financial anxiety, protect your savings, and maintain independence in your later years.

Most importantly, be realistic about aging. Life can turn in a heartbeat. Most of us make the following assumptions:

+ We'll remain healthy indefinitely.

+ The government will provide for us, if we don't.

+ Our money will last our lifetime.

+ Our families will be our caregivers.

+ Our spouses will have plenty of money left when we're gone.

These assumptions are not realistic or practical, so consider the following for your later years:

+ If you become disabled or unable to care for yourself, how will it impact you and your family?

+ What is your desired quality of life?

+ Do you want to remain independent and choose to live where you want?

Steps you can take

+ Have a financial care plan: be sure to incorporate the cost of care into your financial plan for retirement. This is often overlooked as we tend to financially plan for a long and healthy lifestyle. Statistics prove this may not be so. Canadians feel the biggest risk to their retirement plan is the unexpected cost of aging. Between an aging population, longer lifespans, and medical advances, there's a growing sense in financial planning that a sound retirement plan must include a way to address the costs of care if you can't look after yourself. Can your retirement plan pass the financial "stress test" in the event of illness or disability? If not, consider long-term care insurance and include it in your financial plan.

+ Take out long-term care insurance. There is no financial product more suited to the times than long-term care insurance. It is an affordable solution. This option will soon be more difficult to obtain. The real cost of care in the future will far exceed the cost of the premiums today. Policies pay out tax-free benefits that can be spent as you require, or they reimburse you for certain costs. Monthly costs in a long-term care home could run from $1,000 to $5,000, which could exceed your planned income and limit your options and quality of care. Too often, people wait until they're too old to buy it when the price becomes unaffordable.

The most common cost of care is a caregiver. Long-term care insurance will cover this expense.

The hidden costs of loss of independence or cognitive impairment can add up. These expenses can be steep, leading you to cash in savings or rely on family for support. Long-term care insurance covers such costs as meals, transportation, home conversion, a monitoring system and equipment purchase or rental.

Many of us believe the government will look after us. This is an unrealistic assumption.

Long-term care insurance is a relatively new concept, easy to obtain and very affordable.

We live with so much anxiety. Let's tackle this one and have peace of mind knowing our later years will be good ones, for ourselves and our loved ones.

Seeing Past the Noise

Melanie Walbridge

> **Peace. It does not mean to be in a place where there is no noise, trouble, or hard work. It means to be in the midst of those things and still be calm in your heart**
> — *Anonymous*

I used to believe that one day I would wake up and life would be perfect. After all, I worked hard and had been through lots of noise and trouble all my life. I deserve it right? To be perfect.

Here's my story.

As a kid I was labeled at-risk. What the heck does at-risk even mean? Risk of what? Safety? I didn't even step on ants as a kid, let alone jeopardize anyone's safety. I was vegetarian and proudly wore my PETA tee-shirt everywhere when I wasn't wearing my "Save the whales" tee. At that time there was an automatic assumption that if I were poor and in a single parent family, I would negatively impact a peer's life by bringing them down and encouraging bad behaviour. I have a fond memory from a Grade 13 (yes, that grade existed at one point) economics class working on a project to reform Canada's welfare system. I was so perplexed by this project. Just looking at numbers alone, white collar crime in Canada far outweighed welfare fraud. I thought, "Why are we going after these guys here when those guys over there are costing us more?" It was at this point I called bullshit on blaming the poor, and decided to become a social worker.

I sought refuge at school through teachers and professors. Though never an A+ student and almost flunking out of my first year of university from partying too hard, I saw the value of education. My teachers and professors seemed to have answers that I longed for. Yes, there was trouble, noise, and hard work, but I focused on that one-day scenario. One day I will wake up and life will all make sense. I persevered.

Damn, I even lived in la-la-land in a fancy condo by the sea, sipping wheatgrass, running marathons, and came home to a beach-blond-beautiful hunk of a beamer-driving man. As I contemplated working on my PhD, noise and trouble occurred again. My father, to whom I was never close, was sick. My hunk had a wandering eye and my work visa was running out. Wait, what had happened to my perfect life?

Leaving my home, relationship, and studies, I spent time with a man that I didn't have a relationship with. I was broken hearted and broke. However, that broken time was one of the most powerful in my life. Through the noise, trouble, and hard work, life started to make sense. My father passed away, but I had got to know the man at his most pressing time and make peace with him. I got to know my siblings through this difficult time. I felt compassion for my mother, understanding that she couldn't be there for me in order to keep us alive.

I learned a powerful lesson that no PhD could have taught me: life will always bring noise, trouble, and hard work, but how you deal with it is what counts. There has to be an acceptance that stress exists, that Monday might suck but Saturday won't be so bad. We can't pretend that one day we will wake up and have life all figured out, as that day will never exist. Anxiety is worry about the future and depression is worry about the past.

We can't compare ourselves to the picture-perfect selfie that someone snaps. We will have bad days that no one snaps. I try to avoid the illusion that one day I will have everything figured out, as there is where anxiety lies. If we live that way, the bar will always be raised higher. Bad days are okay, and it is okay to throw ourselves a bone once in awhile.

Don't believe it? Look into numerous spiritual practices. When Buddha says embrace suffering, this isn't a downer. This is a direct reference to acknowledging that stress/anxiety will always exist, but how we deal with it is what counts. Christ says to "Not worry about tomorrow and tomorrow will worry about itself" (Matthew 6.34). Whatever spiritual tradition you celebrate, I encourage you to delve into this topic further. If a spiritual tradition is not your thing, that is fine too. Pre-Socratic Greek philosopher Heraclitus stated, "Everything flows and nothing abides, everything gives way and nothing stays fixed."

Religion was a frightening thought at one point in my life. I felt that some interpretations were judgmental and harsh, that somehow anger and bitterness were okay. I sought peace and comfort in a higher power. Shortly after my father's funeral I was ordering an Americano at a local café and noticed someone wearing a tee-shirt with the verse, "Be Still and Know that I am God." That was so powerful for me: through the noise of life I know that there is someone or something joining me in peace and love. This, from a book I once viewed as harsh and critical.

The verse remains a consistent thought in my mind. In fact, something as simple as reminding myself of it in a difficult circumstance helps me let go of the anxiety I may be experiencing. I have also found that, when anxious, I would constantly focus on the future. When feeling depressed I would focus on the past. Recognizing that the only control I had was over the present time has helped me to lesson anxious and depressing thoughts.

I remember going to yoga classes for about a week. I felt great in both body and mind. My body felt toned and strong, but also my mind was able to let things go a little more easily, as that is what the instructor encouraged. She would end sessions with "Namaste and go in peace." During those classes I was often positioned beside a woman who may have embraced only half of the teaching. She was beautiful to watch as she did all yoga poses in complete perfection and had an incredibly toned body. However, she only embraced the physical part of yoga and not the mental part. I witnessed this same woman in the community struggling with anger, whether it was raising her voice at a barista to hurry it up with her coffee or honking at others to get out of the way. Clearly she had not embraced "go in peace." That is why it is important to recognize these and move to change your mind to a better place.

It is important to shift your focus to maintaining peace in your heart instead of focusing on the noise, trouble, and hard work. Sounds like a Hallmark card, right? Take a small example. Someone cuts you off while you're driving. You can choose to focus on that bad driver all day, or you can choose to focus on where you are driving to. This isn't ignoring the fact that there is noise and trouble in the world. There will always be bad drivers. But you can deal with them and move on. You are safe, no one got hurt. Focus on being thankful for that and on your destination. The only way to do this is through the thoughts you think. Thoughts need exercise just like your body, in recognizing them but also in changing them.

Anxiety will always be lingering around trying to get your attention and distract you. Don't ignore it; it exists for a reason, but just learn to handle it in a different way. Remain calm in your heart.

Senjutsu of Chikara Warriors

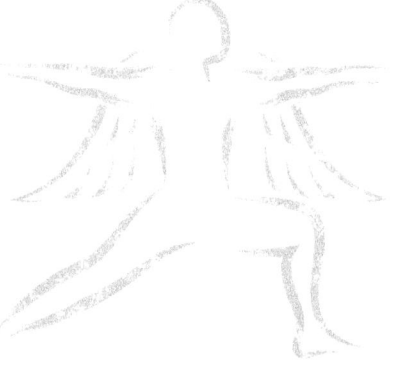

Senjutsu (tactics) of the Chikara Warriors

The Chikara Warriors have many varied strengths and tools, and I am certain I have missed some in the listings. They showed me the consistent combination that got them through their obstacles. Along with *awareness* and *daily practice,* the other common senjutsu from the Chikara Warrior Stories are *courage,* the *determination* to overcome obstacles in their lives, and *to believe they can thrive.* You, the reader already have courage, it took courage to open this book and read it this far. I am certain you have a story too.

Also, they are all dedicated and give of themselves, a great service to help others.

**Helping others and adding value to their lives
gives purpose and value to one's own life.**

✦ Awareness

✦ Daily practice

✦ Courage

✦ Determination

✦ The belief that thriving is possible

✦ Service to others

A Different Kind of Warrior Now — Kathryn Boland

✧ animal therapy
✧ education/research
✧ medication
✧ physical activity

✧ positive self-talk
✧ reaching out
✧ yoga

Anxiety Can Lead You Further — Barb Campbell

- connecting with others
- letting emotions flow
- listening to music that inspires you
- physical activity
- practicing self-responsibility
- prayer, meditation
- reaching out for therapeutic support
- using healthy distractions to change channels, vacation from your troubles

The Miracle of Pets — Sarah Clifford

- animal therapy
- introspection
- self-advocacy
- self-care

Work Anxiety — Magdalene Carson

- introspection
- metaphors
- mindfulness meditation
- positive self-talk

A Moment Can Change a Life — Angie Davis

- acceptance
- meditation
- metaphors
- physical activity
- positive self-talk
- yoga

I'll Be Fine — Amanda Duncan

- authenticity, being true to oneself
- partnering with the brain, being the boss of your brain
- positive self-talk
- reaching out for help
- reaching out to EAP (Employment Assistance Program)
- self-advocacy
- yoga, relaxation

Couples Experience: His and Her Viewpoints — Amanda and Noel Duncan

- connection
- embracing vulnerability
- introspection
- reaching out for help

When Anxiety Encounters Traditional Chinese Medicine — Kory Sadie Ford

- communication skills
- determination
- education/research
- emotional release
- moderation
- nutrition
- physical activity
- self-talk

The Masks We Wear — Karen Girard

- education
- reaching out
- self-care
- self-advocacy

House of Cards to Happiness — Tracey Howarth

- animal therapy
- introspection
- medication
- physical exercises
- reaching out for help
- self-care
- self-talk

Pushing Through My Diagnosis — Meaghan O'Neill

- connection
- distraction/brain shift
- nature
- physical exercise
- reaching out
- self-acceptance

I Got This: Unlocking Your Instincts — Nancy Osborne

- choice to give to others
- connections
- education
- gratitude
- introspection
- passion

A Caregiver's Chronicle — M. Secord

- connection
- introspection
- self-advocacy
- showing up

Seeing Past the Noise — Melanie Walbridge

- education
- introspection
- physical activity
- spiritual practice
- yoga

A Mental Checklist

In my personal life, as well as in my professional practice, I have learned that I need to check in with myself — my body, mind, spirit, and emotions. When I have anxiety, I start working through a mental checklist of possible anxiety triggers.

For instance, I've learned that if I wake up with anxiety, it could be a sign of dehydration. If this is the case, within minutes of drinking water the anxious feeling goes away.

If the anxiety persists, I begin looking at what is on my schedule. Too many things to do? Stress-related events? Deadlines? Something exciting?

To reduce the anxiety, I do some grounding exercises, such as slower breathing, or perhaps take a walk or do some yoga. I also begin some self-talk and journaling. These are just some of the items on my personal list of strategies. Sometimes I need to resort to essential oils such as lavender and frankincense (page 97).

My mental checklist

I've reproduced my mental checklist below. Start one for yourself. First, ask yourself, what are my symptoms? Headaches, tense shoulders, localized pain, nausea, shaking, heart pain?

+ Is the cause physical?

+ Have I slept enough?

+ Do I need water?

+ Is the cause a substance? What did I ingest? What did I eat yesterday?

+ Is the cause external?

✦ Am I wearing my proper glasses? (Sometimes I wear magnifiers.)

✦ Am I excited? Sometimes I am so excited my body feels anxious.

✦ What is on my agenda? Have I piled far too many things on myself? Has life?

✦ What are my thoughts; kind and loving, or critical?

✦ Am I over stimulated?

When asking myself these questions, I'm really working through the eleven layers of anxiety described earlier (pages 26 to 36). It's a helpful starting point for creating your own mental checklist.

Supportive Charts

Chart #1

Start writing a simple list of the things that you enjoy, and that just make you feel good. Lists are good to have handy — they are especially supportive when we are tired . . . too weary to think clearly to the next step. Turning to such tools when times are tough or when you are feeling low or insecure can help to renew your energy and lift your mood.

The following is part of my support list. Create your own list under these headings:

SPIRITUAL	PHYSICAL	EMOTIONAL	MENTAL	SENSUAL
Meditation	Bike riding	Hugs	Study	Lovely clothes
Nia	Snowshoeing	Cooking	Movies	Essential oils
Singing	Dancing	Time with my children	Reading	Dance
Reading inspirational text	Fresh air	My dog		
Gratitude list	Sunshine			
Long walks	Hiking			
Breathing exercises	Organic food			
	Supplements			

Chart #2

I designed this chart to include things I regularly do, as well as things I want more support on. Occasionally, I modify the chart.

The more checks I have, the better I feel. Awarding myself check marks helps me to include more positive things in my life, and even to trim off a few pounds. For each chart I complete, I give myself a reward.

Whenever I find myself getting worn down and tired or feeling overwhelmed, then I know it's time to pull out this chart. It quickly lets me know what I've been neglecting. Below is my own example, but you can create your own categories.

Every day, "feed" all aspects of yourself, including your spiritual, emotional, mental, physical and sensual aspects.

SUPPORTIVE CHART															
Morning stretch															
Breathing															
Journal writing															
Gratitude list															
A walk															
Other exercise															
Taking a rest															
Spiritual reading															
Humming, singing															
Sunshine															
Hugs															
Fun															
Healthy snacks, apples															
More veggies															
Evening stretch															

Another part of my daily practice

In *Anxiety Warrior Volume One*, I shared my daily practice and elements in my biography, and included many support tools for you, the reader, to build your own daily practice. I continue to grow in this practice and add to it. The questions below have further enhanced my life.

In this exercise, take your time to answer. I have these questions in my journal and over time fill in the answers as I notice my body energy lift. The answers are clues, not absolutes for the direction of a life you love to be in.

What centres you?

To be centred takes desire, commitment, time, and practice. Do you know what it feels like to be centred? Perhaps life has been so fast, busy, and chaotic that the feelings of being grounded and centred are unknown. Learn to tell the difference. We know the feeling of stress and of feeling unbalanced.

Try to be centred, calm, quiet, peaceful, at ease, feeling soft. Perhaps it is sitting in nature, yoga, connecting to your body. Is it while walking in nature, listening to music, perhaps being in prayer, or breathing and meditating, or being mindful?

Learn where your centredness is, then go there often. From your place of centredness, here are further questions to contemplate and explore:

Who and what enhances your life?

- ✦ *Who does it feel good to be around?*
- ✦ *What activities make you feel better?*
- ✦ *What forms of nature speak to your soul?*
- ✦ *What opens your heart?*
- ✦ *What helps you feel alive?*
- ✦ *What breathes life into your spirit?*
- ✦ *What revitalizes you?*

What refreshes you, renews you, or pumps you up?

Create the life you love to look at. Bring excitement into your intention.

Set a new tone to life, let your heart send energy into your day, into your life.

Empowering
Your Own Anxiety Warrior

Initially, if I could only give you two words from this book, they would be *awareness* and *practice*.

**Become aware so you know what to change/
modify/manage and practice in your strategies.**

Life is a process and a practice for all of us!

The Chikara Warriors show us many varied strengths and tools, and how, by consistently combining them, the warriors overcame their obstacles. With *awareness, daily practice, courage,* and *determination,* they came to believe that thriving was possible. You, the reader already have courage, it took courage to open this book and read it this far. I am certain you have a story too.

Also, they all dedicate of themselves, a great service to help others.

**By adding value to others and helping
others there is purpose value in life.**

✦ Awareness

✦ Daily practice

✦ Courage

✦ Determination

✦ The belief that thriving is possible

✦ Service to others

No matter what type of anxiety you're dealing with, anxiety can be managed by the following strategies:

✦ Begin with a mental checklist (page 290).

✦ Explore and understand the possibility of a specific type of anxiety.

✦ Accept your anxiety as a gift, a signal, an opportunity, a message.

✦ Identify and understand the causes and triggers for your anxiety.

✦ Use the scale 0 to 10 to identify the intensity of your anxiety.

✦ Know your limits (sleep, hunger, amount and type of stressors).

✦ Perhaps break down your anxiety into smaller layers.

✦ Manage the easy layers first, right away.

✦ Change your lifestyle to lower your anxiety.

✦ Practice your strategies.

✦ Create your own daily practice and practice it daily, especially when you feel pleasant.

As you have read, there are many facets to anxiety. It is more than just a word or condition. Anxiety can be a gift, an opportunity inviting us to look deeper into ourselves. I hope that you have found inspiration to explore and sooth those tender parts of yourself.

I used to curse anxiety and its symptoms. I hated it! I tried to tame it, chase it away with a stick or a song. I thought it was weak and sick. When I began to be curious, I cautiously ventured closer to it, to try and understand it. As I explored anxiety, it showed me myself and my life. I learned about the vulnerable part of me, that was worthy of love and kindness and of thriving. I hope this book has gently opened some doors for your curiosity.

You are worth it! We can do this!

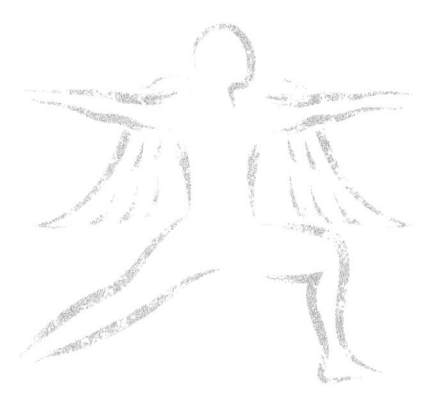

Glossary

AMYGDALA: Almond-shaped structure adjoined to the temporal lobe of the brain's limbic system. It is responsible for detecting fear, regulating emotions, and preparing the body to respond to danger.

ANXIETY: A state of worry, nervousness, or unease, typically about an imminent event or something with an uncertain outcome. A feeling of concern, apprehension, unease, fearfulness, disquiet, agitation, angst, tension, twitchiness, or nervousness. Mostly felt in anticipation of something happening. It is a natural alarm response that helps people avoid dangerous situations and is a signal to motivate them to solve everyday problems.

ANXIETY DISORDER: Anxiety disorders are mental health problems characterized by excessive levels of alarm, fear, or worry due to anticipated or perceived danger. They significantly interfere with day-to-day living. There are many different types of anxiety disorders, including bipolar disorder and depressive disorder (depression).

ASSERTIVENESS: When people act in their own best interests without manipulating or harming others. When people exercise their right of self- expression without denying the rights of others.

BELIEFS: Beliefs are firm opinions or convictions. Belief systems are a set of beliefs or principles that characterize a community, religion, or philosophy. They are often influenced by culture, which in turn guides behaviour and communication. Cultural belief systems can shape a person's understanding of health and illness.

BIPOLAR DISORDER: Bipolar disorder is a type of mood disorder in which a person alternates between states of clinical depression and mania. Bipolar disorder is sometimes called manic depression.

COMMUNITY MENTAL HEALTH TEAM (CMHT): CMHTs look after the welfare of people who need more attention to their mental health problems than a family doctor can provide. Care teams vary from area to area and can include psychiatrists, psychologists, community psychiatric nurses, social workers, housing and welfare officers.

COGNITION: Thinking, understanding, and learning.

DEFENSIVE PESSIMISM: Defensive pessimism is a strategy of imagining worst-case scenarios. Anxious people use this to help them work productively. When practicing this method, expectations are lowered so that there is less likelihood of disappointment. This may sound depressing, though it helps some people distract themselves enough to function and work.

DELUSIONS: Delusions are fixed, false beliefs that are not culturally sanctioned. They may arise from distorted interpretations of reality. They may include beliefs of persecution, guilt, having a special mission, or being under outside control. No matter how bizarre the delusions may seem to others, the people experiencing them believe they are real.

DEPRESSIVE DISORDER (DEPRESSION): Depression is characterized by either a sad or irritable mood, or the loss of interest or enjoyment in nearly all activities for a period of at least two weeks. Depression is more than short-term feelings of sadness.

EMDR: This stands for Eye Movement Desensitization and Reprocessing, though it does not have much to do with the eyes. This therapy uses bi-lateral movement stimulation in which eyes move back and forth, or bi-lateral body movement, like tapping or wearing a headset using alternating beeps or music.

EMDR was developed in the late 80s in the US and was primarily used for war veterans with Post Traumatic Stress Disorder (PTSD). It has quickly come to be useful in eliminating all the symptoms associated with stress and trauma, like flashbacks, panic attacks, intrusive thoughts, anxiety, phobias, depression, over-reactive anger, worrying, disturbed sleep, and so on. It has been studied and validated all around the world.

Sometimes, memories get stuck in the information processing system of the brain, along with pictures, sounds, smells, tastes, emotions, and bodily sensations, which were all part of the original experience. When memories are stuck, this is where EMDR 'desensitizes and reprocesses' the memory, helping the brain reprocess the memory, to a point where remembering the event no longer causes distress and the sufferer has peace with it.

Research has not yet shown how the brain files memories during EMDR. It is similar to the dream stage, or Rapid Eye Movement (REM) stage of sleep. EMDR may be a kind of accelerated, conscious version of REM sleep.

EMDR is approved as an evidence-based, best-practice trauma therapy for PTSD and related issues by many international health and government bodies, including the World Health Organization (WHO) in 2013, the American Psychological Association (APA) in 2004 and 2009, and the American Department of Defense/Veterans' Affairs (2004 and 2010).

EMOTIONAL FREEDOM: Emotional freedom means leading a joyful life. The body feels a full range of emotions and is able to understand and process them.

EMOTIONAL HIJACKING: This occurs when the mind feels like it is being hijacked by an emotion. This occurs in an instant and before the brain is able to fully grasp the situation and the reaction.

EMOTIONAL INTELLIGENCE: Emotional intelligence means having a skill set to deal with emotions in a useful way. It is the ability to motivate ourselves, regulate our moods, and control impulses/reactions.

FEAR: Fear happens when something threatens a person, while worry is being afraid in anticipation of something happening. They both have the same physiological response in the body. For example, fear is when you are in the woods and a bear chases you. You are afraid, you must make a decision, you must run or take cover. Fear is an important human emotion. It has kept the human race alive.

MANIA: Mania is one of the emotional extremes associated with bipolar disorder. Mania is characterized by an elevated mood, grandiose ideas, and irritability for a period of at least one week. Mania usually starts suddenly and can increase rapidly over a few days.

MASLOW'S HIERARCHY: Maslow's hierarchy of needs is usually depicted like the triangle below. In 1943, American psychologist Abraham Maslow was curious about what motivated humans. He surmised that the most basic physiological needs for survival were the most important, such as air, shelter, warmth, water, food, and rest. It is important to feel secure and safe, to have protection from the elements, and to have a sense of stability. These are the most fundamental and crucial needs. As shown in the illustration, love, belonging, and self-esteem are also considered to be basic needs.

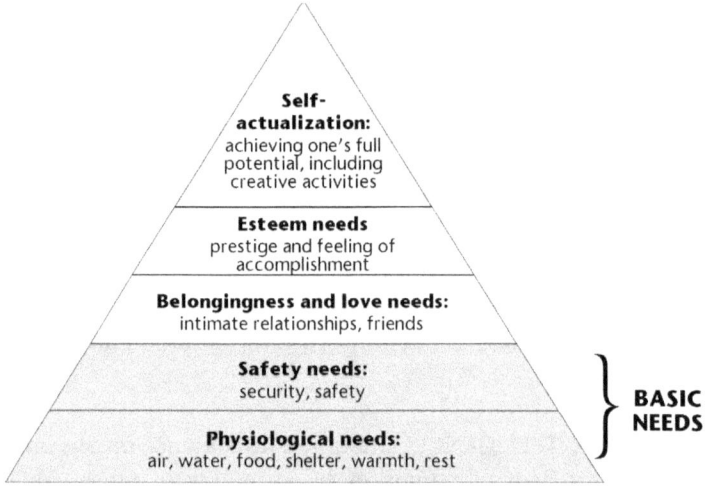

Maslow's theory was that when humans had their basic needs met, then they could progress to higher goals such as self-actualization, self-fulfillment, and achievement. His research showed that as the quality of their needs rose, so did the quality of their activities, production and creativity.

If humans need to struggle to meet basic needs of survival, or if these needs are not met, humans experience stress, tension, uncertainty, fear, and anxiety.

MENTAL DISORDER: A mental disorder causes major changes in a person's thinking, emotional state, and behaviour, and disrupts a person's ability to work and to carry out normal personal relationships.

MENTAL HEALTH: Mental health is a state of well-being in which individuals realize their own abilities, can cope with the normal stresses of life, can work productively, and are able to make a contribution to their community.

MENTAL HEALTH PROBLEM: A mental health problem is a broad term that includes both mental disorders and symptoms that may not be severe enough to warrant the diagnosis of a mental disorder.

MOOD DISORDER: Mood disorders are mental health problems characterized by disturbances in the way a person feels and experiences emotion, and which make it difficult for the person to function in day-to-day life.

PATHOLOGICAL ANXIETY: The psychiatric meaning is a nervous disorder characterized by a state of excessive uneasiness and apprehension, typically with compulsive behaviour or panic attacks. When anxiety is a problem it affects our health, our well-being and our happiness. When anxiety stops us from doing something, like going out of the house, going shopping, driving, taking a course, going to a party, or visiting family, it is a problem.

PREMENSTRUAL SYNDROME (PMS) refers to physical and emotional symptoms that occur in the one to two weeks before a woman's period. Symptoms often vary between women and resolve around the start of bleeding. Common symptoms include acne, tender breasts, bloating, feeling tired, irritability, and mood changes.

PSYCHIATRIST: Psychiatrists are medical doctors who specialize in mental health and mental illness. Psychiatrists make diagnoses, decisions about treatment and care, and prescribe psychiatric drugs and therapies.

PSYCHOLOGIST: Psychologists study the human mind and its effects on behaviour. Psychologists can use behaviour therapy to help people work through the way they act in certain situations.

SELF-ESTEEM: Self-esteem is the way we feel about ourselves and our abilities and reflects the value we place on ourselves as human beings.

SELF-STIGMA: The prejudice and discrimination people face because of mental health problems often become internalized. People with mental health problems begin to believe the negative things that other people and the media say about them. They have lower self-esteem because they feel guilt and shame. As a result, they often do not seek the help they need.

STIGMA: Stigma refers to negative attitudes (prejudices) and negative behaviours (discrimination) toward people who have problems with substance abuse and/or mental health. Stigma means having fixed ideas and making judgments about people, as well as feeling disgust and avoiding what isn't understood. Stigma results in the exclusion of people with mental health problems from activities that are open to other people, such as getting a job, finding a safe place to live, participating in social activities, and having relationships.

STIMULANTS: Caffeine has a directly stimulating effect on several different systems in the body. Too much caffeine can keep a person in a tense, aroused condition, leaving one more vulnerable to generalized anxiety as well as panic attacks. For those people who are very sensitive to caffeine, less than 50 mg/day is advisable.

Nicotine is as strong a stimulant as caffeine. It stimulates increased physiological arousal and makes the heart work harder. People who smoke are more prone to anxiety states and panic.

STRESS: Stress is a demand on physical or mental energy that may or may not disturb a person's normal functioning.

References

A Course in Miracles. The Foundation for Inner Peace, Viking, New York, NY, 1996. *(A non-denominational book on God, Jesus, and living. A very dense book, best studied with groups.)*

Allen, James. *As a Man Thinketh.* Thomas Y. Crowell Co., New York, NY, 1902.

Attwood, Janet, and Chris Attwood, *The Passion Test, The Effortless Path to Discovering Your Life Purpose,* Penguin Books, New York, NY, 2007.

Balch, Phyllis, A, CNC, Prescription for Nutritional Healing, Avery, New York, NY, 2000. *(This book is updated regularly, watch for the newest edition.)*

Bassett, Lucinda. *From Panic to Power,* HarperCollins, New York, NY, 1997. *(Easy to read; the author uses many of her personal experiences in a humorous way. Included are many support points for anxiety and worry.)*

Benson, Herbert. *The Relaxation Response.* William Morrow and Company, New York, NY, 1975.

Bourne, Edmund PhD, *The Anxiety and Phobia Workbook,* New Harbinger Publications, Oakland, CA, 2015.

Bilodeau, Lorraine. *The Anger Workbook.* Hazelden Foundation, Center City, MN, 1994. *(A simple workbook designed to get the reader thinking and understanding, and to help the reader redirect feelings of frustration and anger.)*

Brown, Brené. *The Gifts of Imperfection.* Hazelden Publishing, Center City, MN, 2010.

Buettner, Dan. *The Blue Zones,* Lessons for living longer from the people who've lived the longest. National Geographic, Washington, DC, 2008.

Cameron, Julia. *The Artist's Way.* Tarcher/Perigee, New York, NY, 1992. *(A 12-week program to help readers discover their creative selves and their creative blocks. Lots of applications; best done with a buddy or in a group.)*

Campbell, Don. *The Mozart Effect.* Avon Books, The Hearst Corporation, New York, NY, 1997.

Canfield, Jack. *The Success Principles*. HarperCollins, New York, NY, 2007.

Chancellor, Philip M., *Illustrated Handbook of the Bach Flowers Remedies*. Hillman Printers, Great Britain, 1971.

Dennison, Paul E., and Gail E. Dennison. *Brain Gym*. Edu-Kinesthetics, Ventura, CA, 1986. *(Many practical exercises to relax, rejuvenate, and stimulate brain activity.)*

Dispenza, Joe. *You Are the Placebo*. Hay House, Carlsbad, CA, 2014. *(This book is about how to make your mind matter in creating your health and your life. It is backed by science and a team of doctors.)*

Ikeda, Daisaku. *Faith into Action*. World Tribune Press, Santa Monica, CA, 1999. *(A collection containing reflections for many life situations. Based on a Buddhist perspective.)*

Doidage, Norman, *The Brain that Changes Itself*, Penguin Books, New York, NY, 2007.

Franck, Frederick. *The Zen of Seeing*, Random House, New York, NY, 1973.

Frankl, Victor, *Man's Search for Meaning*, Washington Square Press, New York, NY, 1984.

Gawain, Shakti. *Creative Visualization: Meditations*. New World Library, Novato, CA, 1995.

Gendlin, Eugene T. *Focusing*, Bantam Books, New York, NY, 1978 and 1982.

Goldberg, Natalie. *Writing Down the Bones*. Shambhala Press, Boston, MA, 1986. *(All her books are excellent guides for stimulating self-discovery through writing.)*

Goldstein, Nathan. *The Art of Responsive Drawing*. Prentice Hall, Upper Saddle River, NJ, 1973.

Goleman, David. *Emotional Intelligence*. Bantam Books, New York, NY, 1995.

Gray, John. *Practical Miracles for Mars and Venus*. HarperCollins, New York, NY, 1999.

Hart, Mickey with Jay Stevens. *Drumming at the Edge of Magic*. HarperCollins, San Francisco, CA, 1960.

Hay, Louise. *You Can Heal Your Life*. Hay House, Carlsbad, CA, 1999.

Heath, Yvonne, *Love Your Life to Death: How to Plan and Prepare for End of Life So You Can Live Fully Now*. Port Sydney, ON, 2015

Jenkinson, Stephen, *How It Could All Be: A work book for dying people and for those that love them*, First Choice Books, Victoria, BC, 2009.

Jeffers, Sue, Dr., *Feel the Fear and Do It Anyway*. Random House, London, UK, 1991.

Kavelin Popov, Linda. *The Family Virtues Guide.* Plume Books, Penguin Group, New York, NY, 1997. (*A basic book about morals and character.*)

Kriz, Jurgen, *Self Actualization*, Germany, Books on Demand, 2006.

Liedloff, Jean. *The Continuum Concept.* Addison-Wesley Publication Co. Inc., Reading, MA, 1985.

May, Rollo. *The Courage to Create.* Norton, New York, NY, 1975.

Murdock, Maureen. *Spinning Inward: guided imagery for children for learning, creativity and relaxation.* Shambala Publications, Boston, MA, 1987.

Nicolaides, Kimon. *The Natural Way to Draw.* Houghton Mifflin Company, Boston, MA, 1969.

Pearson, Carol. *The Hero Within.* HarperCollins, New York, NY, 1991. (*Various human characteristics illustrated using hero characters.*)

Peck, M. Scott. *The Road Less Travelled.* Simon & Schuster, New York, NY, 1978.

Pitman, Walter, Ontario Arts Council. *Making the Case for Arts Education.* Ontario Arts Council, Toronto, ON, 1997.

Pearce, Joseph. *Magical Child.* Penguin Group, New York, NY, 1997.

Rinpoche, Sogyal. *The Tibetan Book of Living and Dying.* HarperOne, San Francisco, CA, 2002.

Rosenberg, Marshall. *The Surprising Purpose of Anger. Beyond Anger Management: Finding the Gift.* PuddleDancer Press. (*Rosenberg won over seven peace awards for his work.*)

Rosenberg, Marshall. *Nonviolent Communication: A Language of Life.* PuddleDancer Press, Encinitas, CA, 2015. (*There are many YouTube videos about this online and he has written many books explaining his model.*)

Roth, Gabrielle. *Maps to Ecstasy: Teachings of an Urban Shaman.* New World Library, San Rafael, CA, 1989.

Shinn, Florence, *Your Word Is Your Wand,* Dotesios Printers Ltd., Essex, UK, 1928.

Shinn, Florence, *The Game of Life*, Essex, UK, Dotesios Dotesios Printers Ltd., 1928.

Sobel, Elliot. *Wild Heart Dancing.* Fireside Press, New York, NY, 1987. (*A self-directed private creativity retreat. To be taken along and only read as you complete exercises. Lots of fun and worthwhile*).

Tavris, Carol. *Anger: the Misunderstood Emotion.* Simon&Schuster, New York, NY, 1982.

Tisserand, Robert B., *The Art of Aromatherapy*, Destiny Books, Rochester, VL, 1977.

Tolle, Eckhart, *Power of Now*, Namaste Publishing, Vancouver, BC, 1997.

Tolle, Eckhart, *A New Earth, Awakening to Your Life's Purpose*, Plume, Penguin Group, New York, NY, 2006.

Von Oech, Roger. *A Whack on the Side of the Head.* Warner Books, New York, NY, 1998.

Zukav, Gary, *The Seat of the Soul.* Shambhala Publications, Boston, MA, 1991.

About the Contributors

Susan Allen—Sat Akal Kaur

Living with her family in Muskoka and running a landscape gardening and native plant nursery business for 40 years, Susan feels a close connection to the earth. Practicing Hatha Yoga and Nia for over 16 years, she trained in mindfulness-based stress reduction in 2009. Susan loves to travel and learn new things. Introduced to Kundalini Yoga by a friend, Susan fell in love with the practice. As Sat Akal Kaur (her spiritual name) she completed Kundalini Yoga Teacher Training Level One, as taught by Yogi Bhajan at PranaShanti Yoga Studio in Ottawa, plus over eight months with Devinder Kaur, in May 2015. In August 2015, Sat Akal began her journey to become a Level Two Kundalini Yoga Practitioner. The curriculum set by the Kundalini Research Institute cannot be completed in less than two years. Sat Akal recently met these requirements.

www.kundaliniyogamuskoka.com for classes and events.

Emma Scholz Bertrand

Emma Scholz Bertrand is in the second semester of her second year at university. For most of her life, she wanted to be a vet. Emma saved her money, worked every summer, and as soon as she could began to save for seven-plus years of university. However, after taking certain courses at university and working at a vet clinic, Emma realized that being a vet was not in line with her values. Her passions are more holistic and encompass not only saving animals, but also people and the environment. This awareness began her journey of discovering her true dreams, and also rediscovering herself.

Emma.L.Scholz@gmail.com

Dr. Nick Bianchi

Dr. Nick Bianchi, B.SC. (KIN), D.C., is a chiropractor, published author, speaker and lecturer practicing in Bracebridge, Ontario. His model of health care and his clinical approach include a whole-person wellness perspective and patient education. Author Elke Scholz is a favorite guest speaker of his patients and of Dr. Nick as well.

> Bracebridge Chiropractic and Wellness Centre, 705-645-9544
> info@bracebridgechiro.com
> www.bracebridgechiro.com

Kathryn Boland

Kathryn Boland is a long-time dancer and yoga practitioner. She is also a Certified Yoga Instructor, with a BA in dance and an MA in expressive therapies, notably dance/movement therapy. In this work, she has served diverse individuals who have myriad needs, desires, and capabilities—from low-income youth to elders with memory disorders. She also is a staff writer for *Yoga U Online* and *Dance Informa Magazine*. She is fascinated by, passionate about, and devoted to spreading the use of movement and creativity to express, heal, and empower. For non-work-related enjoyment, Kathryn treasures coffee chats with good friends, music, comedy, and time in nature.

> Kdbyoga1@gmail.com

Barbara Campbell

Born and raised in Bracebridge, Ontario, Barb has raised three daughters and has seven grandkids. They are her world. She loves to be called Mom and Nana. Barb followed in her mother's footsteps by going into the healthcare field. She worked in a hospital and nursing home for 37 years. Now retired, Barb continues to have a drive for compassion, respect, love, and confidentially for young and old. She has ridden the Big Bike several times for the Heart and Stroke Foundation, and has volunteered in schools, church, a hospital gift shop, the Royal Canadian Legion, and a nursing home.

Magdalene Carson

Magdalene Carson is a graphic artist based in Ottawa who has specialized in book design for the past 15 years under her company name, New Leaf Publication Design. Making art and objects throughout her youth, she eventually pursued art as a means to enhance life in society. She completed a three-year program, *Architectural Art: Art for Public Places*, at Fanshawe College in London, Ontario. Her working life has always been in the fields of art, design, printing, and publishing. Curiosity and passion about ideas, cultures, and all things human has taken her down many sideroads; for example, she has travelled widely, from the Orkney Islands to Egypt and from India to Cuba, and has participated in a number of social and political projects. Magdalene feels that this combined experience has lent her the skill to connect with the unique story of each author and find its expression in a fitting design solution.

www.newleafpublicationdesign.ca
magcar@rogers.com

Sarah Clifford

Sarah Clifford has been a paramedic in Muskoka for over 16 years. She received her diploma in the paramedic program in 2001 from Northern College in Timmins and passed her provincial testing soon after graduation. She volunteers with the Chief Ceremonial Unit at her workplace, with the therapy dog program in Muskoka, and with the Ontario Mounted Special Services Unit. She is a longtime resident of Gravenhurst, Ontario, where she lives with her husband and two children. Her passions include spending time with family and friends, riding her horses, walking her dogs, camping, boating, and traveling.

Dr. Roxanne Daleo

Renowned clinician, leader, and pioneer in health psychology, "Dr. Roxie" has an unwavering passion for helping children discover their inner resources and realize their self-worth. She is a counselor in pediatric stress management, specializing in both anxious children and parent coaching. Her training from Harvard University and the Jung Institute combine evidence-based mind/body techniques with expressive arts, and anchors her work in one of the most powerful methods for awakening natural healing. Dr. Roxie's groundbreaking work as founder of MindWorks for Children provides parents, caregivers, and children with alternative solutions to alleviate stress and anxieties. Her use of art, music, guided imagery, and meditation programs allows children to access their own internal source of strength, love, and innate gifts. She serves on the Board of Directors of the International Expressive Arts Therapy Association.

www.drroxannedaleo.com

Angie Davis

Angie Davis is fueled by a deep desire to be of service to those who are on a healing journey. She is a registered 200-hour yoga teacher and a Trauma Sensitive Yoga Teacher, certified through the Trauma Center at the Justice Resource Institute in Massachussets. She is also a Level 1 iRest Yoga Nidra teacher, accredited by the Integrative Restoration Institute in California. She teaches this research-based, complementary therapy, which has been proven helpful for PTSD, anxiety, sleep difficulties, and other issues. Angie is also trained in Mental Health Sensitivity, Mental Health First Aid, and SafeTALK Suicide Alert Helper. In her career as an elementary school teacher, she is on the Mental Health Steering Committee for Trillium Lakelands District School Board and presents provincially on topics of health and wellness.

angiedavis.ca
info@angiedavis.ca
Instagram as angiedavis

Chantelle Denstedt

Having worked in the fast-paced world of information technology for over 25 years, Chantelle Denstedt sees and experiences her fair share of anxiety and stress. And unfortunately, with technology, the pace and the demands continually get faster. Chantelle has had a strong belief in natural, plant based, and holistic therapies since her teens, when she started reading self-help books and studying natural healing in other parts of the world. When she was introduced to essential oils, she became hooked and has incorporated them into every part of her life. At the same time, Chantelle has been studying how the toxins in our households impact our health, not only on a physical level, but also on an emotional level. She offers classes on how to incorporate essential oils into everyday routines, to support a healthier, less toxic life.

https://www.myyl.com/chantelledenstedt
https://www.instagram.com/be.you.yl/ (@be.you.yl)
cdenstedt2@vianet.ca

Craig Denstedt

Says Craig, "My family moved to Muskoka in 1970 and I spent the first seven years of my life living above a bar. I grew up in the small village of Milford Bay and went to Monck Public school in Bracebridge. I found my calling when I was 13, with the Muskoka Aquatic Club, and over the next seven years I became a nationally ranked swimmer. After my swimming career ended, I got involved in my family's construction business—for the next 25 years. I decided in 2010 to move in a different direction with my life and walked away from the family business. After discovering a passion for tea, I made the big decision to take a chance on opening a retail store in Bracebridge, and it has been one of the best experiences of my life."

Tea Infusion (705) 640-8327
www.teainfusion.ca
www.facebook.com/teainfusion.ca
https://www.instagram.com/teainfusiontea/

Krystal Demaine

Krystal Demaine, PhD, is a Board Certified Music Therapist (MT-BC), Registered Expressive Arts Therapist (REAT), and Registered Yoga Teacher (RYT). She currently holds positions as Associate Professor of Expressive Therapies at Endicott College and Adjunct Faculty at Lesley University in Boston, MA. She has over 15 years of private clinical practice in music therapy. Her professional scholarship and research have included study on music and the brain, east-west perspectives of creative arts therapy, and topics on creative compassion and pedagogy. Krystal enjoys writing, yoga-ing, traveling, playing, and being creative with friends. She lives in Beverly, MA, USA with her son Ezra and their dog Sage.

www.krystaldemaine.com

Amanda Duncan

Amanda was born in the small town of Smiths Falls, Ontario on September 3, 1980. After moving to Muskoka she met the love of her life, Noel. In 2004, they married by the falls on Lake Muskoka. In 2006 they had their first and only child Preston. Amanda has pursued a career in healthcare. She twice graduated with honours from Georgian College, Muskoka Campus by obtaining her personal support worker certificate and later her Practical Nursing Diploma. While completing her diploma program she battled cervical cancer, which changed her life forever. Through the tools she has been taught by great mentors, Amanda continues to be true to herself and to allow room for personal growth. Her biggest accomplishment to date is being a devoted mother to her wonderful philanthropist son Preston. Amanda currently works as an RPN Coordinator for the Victorian Order of Nurses (VON) Canada, where she coordinates daily operations of the VON Assisted Living Service Program for North Durham.

Noel Duncan

Noel Duncan was born in Orillia, Ontario, and raised in the rural village of Washago. His family cottage, built by his grandparents, brought the family there in the 1940s. His parents, Al and Pat, settled close by in the 1970s, where they raised Noel and his younger brother Colin. From an early age Noel was inspired by many kinds of music and in his teens took to writing and performing. While in his early 20s and living with his band in Barrie, Ontario, Noel met the love of his life, Amanda. Inspired by her love of life and dedication to family, they married in 2004 and became parents to their son Preston Woodworth Duncan in 2006. Helping his wife through the process of fighting and beating cancer, while raising their son together, deepened his appreciation for life and how precious every moment can be.

Kory Sadie Ford

Kory Sadie Ford holds an Honours in Biological Science, is a Registered Acupuncturist, Registered Traditional Chinese Medicine Practitioner, Fitness Instructor Specialist, and Personal Trainer Specialist, and Certified Foot Reflexologist. She resides in Guelph, Ontario. Sadie is a self-professed body nerd, always continuing to learn and grow. After being away from Guelph for almost a decade, Sadie is happy to be back planting roots in the community. She fills her time sharing various body movement modalities (yoga, Pilates, group fitness) with others. When she is not teaching movement, you will find her at the clinic. She facilitates others in recognizing themselves as whole beings and mini-ecosystems. This allows reflection on the different components of the self, as well as on how our individual ecosystems interact with the larger ecosystems of the family, the community, and the world. Her goal is to empower and support those around her, allowing them to find their paths on their own unique journeys.

Dr. Colette Harman

In her over 25 years of naturopathic medical practice, Dr. Colette Harman has successfully treated many people suffering from anxiety and depression. She has written the eBook, *Anxiety and Depression: Six Simple Steps to Effectively Cope*, based on her workshops of the same name, in which she has distilled her knowledge of treating anxiety and depression into six simple steps that are easy to learn and implement. As someone who has suffered from both anxiety and depression in her life, Dr. Colette Harman can attest to the effectiveness of these techniques from both a personal and a professional perspective. In short, they work. Based on mindfulness techniques and the power of harnessing the Law of Attraction, Dr. Harman developed these six effective steps to reduce and even eliminate both anxiety and depression.
www.HarmanyWellnessSolutions.com, where you can purchase her eBooks and read her blogs.

Karen Girard

As a passionate career life coach, Karen Girard reduces stress and offers unbiased support and guidance, moving her clients through the steps needed to rediscover their passions and design a life they will be excited to wake up to. She is an Advanced Certified Passion Test Facilitator, with over 20 years' experience in Human Resources and career development, and seven years' experience in developing and presenting workshops. Karen is the founder and principal of Design My Best Life (http://www.designmybestlife.com) and Career Planning for Students, companies specializing in helping people to become successful by learning to live their passions, both at work and in their everyday life. Karen believes that everyone has the power to change their lives by reframing thinking, and that discovering unexplored passions can guide this change. If you are ready to take a leap of faith, contact Karen and ask her for a free 30-minute exploratory session.

Karen@karengirard.ca

http://www.karengirard.com

Tracey Howarth

Tracey Howarth is a retired paramedic and full-time student studying massage therapy. She is also a certified equine massage therapist growing her equine massage therapy practice in Muskoka. Tracey is the owner and author of chickymedic.com, a blog dedicated to creating awareness surrounding PTSD and mental health in first responders. Her post "No, I didn't know," went viral in December 2015 and was published in Canadian Paramedicine Magazine. When not studying or writing, Tracey spends her time with her husband and daughter. They live on a 90-acre property in beautiful Muskoka, with their two horses and Labrador retriever, Piper.

Nicki Koethner

Nicki Koethner, MA, MFT is an Expressive Arts Psychotherapist, Consultant and Educator and Multi-Media Artist. In her practice, she is devoted to playfulness, joy, embodied earth-based spirituality, wholesome sexuality and transforming trauma into empowerment through creativity. She has a private practice in German and English in Berkeley. She is adjunct faculty at Sofia University, California Institute of Integral Studies (CIIS), and supervisor of Art of Health and Healing at the Contra Costa County Health Services (CCHS).

www.express-explore-expand.com

nkoethnermft@yahoo.com

Susan O'Connell

Susan O'Connell is a faculty member at Sofia University, California, where she teaches creative expression, ecopsychology, and spiritual psychology. She has been ordained as an earth-based multicultural minister. She was awarded a professional credential as a Registered Expressive Arts Consultant/Educator (REACE) through the International Expressive Arts Therapy Association (IEATA). She is a co-chair of the REACE professional standards committee with IEATA. She earned a Master's Degree from the Institute of Transpersonal Psychology with a focus in spiritual psychology, ecopsychology and creative expression. Her undergraduate degree from the University of California Santa Barbara, focused on earth and atmospheric science. She has an extensive background in public service leadership. Her interests lie in creative expression, ecopsychology, sacred ecology, and psycho-spiritual development and transformation across the lifespan. She loves nature writing and photography, yoga, hiking, and music.

susan.oconnell@sofia.edu

Meagan O'Neill

Meagan O'Neill lives in Muskoka. She enjoys outdoor activities, including hiking, backpacking, camping, swimming, snowshoeing, and walking her dog. She also enjoys adventuring in places that are less traveled and seeking out the hidden gems that the bush has to offer. Meagan loves animals and has multiple pets in her home. She grew up studying music with the Royal Conservatory of Music, plays the piano, and has studied vocals. She appreciates the time she is able to spend with family.

Nancy Osborne

Nancy Osborne is the recipient of the Canadian Forces Decoration for long service and good conduct. She is founder of I GOT THIS, has more than 30 years' experience as a speaker and trainer, and has presented to audiences around the globe from Afghanistan to New York. At 17, she joined the Canadian Forces as one of the first women in a previously male-only branch. This began many years of being the first, and often only, woman in some of the biggest boys' clubs in the world. After retiring from the military, she was recruited by the United Nations to provide security risk analysis and access negotiations for humanitarian operations in some of the most dangerous and culturally misogynistic places in the world. Nancy attributes her successes to her "I Got This" attitude and listening to her instincts. Over the years she has developed collaborative tactics to overcome the challenges that confront women everywhere. Her stories inspire others to make their presence undeniable and their voices resonate.

http://nancyosborne.ca
https://www.igotthis.space
https://www.linkedin.com/in/nancy-osborne-igotthis/
https://m.facebook.com/unlockingyourinstincts/

Rosscoe Marks

Rossoe Marks's duties at Common Sense Natural Products, the producers of Maté Factor yerba maté teas, are vast and varied. They include production management, logistics and supply, quality assurance, and sales and marketing. He has been with this company since the summer of 2012. Please visit the website, www.matefactor.ca, to learn more about the products and the company.

Reilly Scott

A deep passion for self-exploration and emotional literacy is the foundation for the outpouring of Reilly Scott's work. Synchronicity is what fuels her mission to call people together, eliciting healing and social change through music and the written word. Over the past decade, Reilly has had the privilege of performing her original music and poetry for audiences throughout Canada and overseas. Her debut album, *Beautiful Unfolding*, showcases her journey as a poet, singer/songwriter, and advocate for healing through the arts. Whether on stage or in workshops as a community arts facilitator, Reilly's creative process inspires and encourages others to connect with their own artistic spirit. Reilly continues to create, live and love in the small town of Kenora, Ontario. *Beautiful Unfolding* is available for purchase on iTunes and Bandcamp, and for streaming on Spotify, Apple Music, and Google Play.

    www.reillyscottmusic.ca
    reillyscottmusic@gmail.com
    http://www.facebook.com/reillyscottmusic
    reillyscottmusic@reillyscottmusic

M. Secord

M. Secord is particularly concerned about the anxiety facing Baby Boomers and their families. Her greatest pride is in her two children and the kind, responsible, and caring people they have grown to be. She loves spending time with family and friends, and volunteers for Muskoka Victim Services, the YWCA, and any initiative that helps end violence against women.

Melanie Walbridge

Melanie Walbridge, MA, CRPO, lives in beautiful Bracebridge, Muskoka, Ontario, with her beloved family. In addition to her work as a registered psychotherapist, the travel and tourism industry is an intricate part of her life. She has a background in dialectical behavioural therapy, multisystemic therapy, brief solution focused, and cognitive behavioural therapy. Strong coffee, goofy pug kisses, flannel pajamas, and exploring a new part of the world bring great joy and happiness to her life.

About the Author

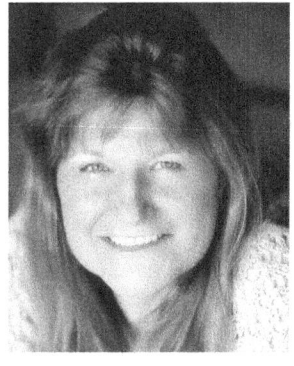

Elke Scholz is a Registered Psychotherapist, a well-known author, therapist, speaker, and facilitator. She was awarded a Masters degree in Expressive Arts Therapy by European Graduate School (EGS), Saas Fee, Switzerland. She is internationally certified in Eye Movement Desensitization and Reprocessing (EMDR) and is a Registered Expressive Arts Consultant/Educator (REACE) with the International Expressive Arts Therapy Association (IEATA).

Elke has been helping people since 1980. Her calm approach invites a comfortable space for people to try new things. Elke can be with clients in their darkest, hardest times. Her acute awareness and high sensitivity are tremendous assets for her clients and make her distinctive in her field. Elke works well with teams of educators, social workers, doctors, corporations, organizations, and groups. Other facilitators immensely enjoy her training sessions and supervision.

All her life, Elke has understood the connection between the arts and living. For her, the elements connect at every level, and she is able to simplify concepts and relay this to other people in a simple, approachable way. Elke communicates this understanding, as well as her own artistic vision, in numerous ways.

Elke's program development work focuses on attachment, grief, trauma, and loss recovery using Expressive Arts. She successfully manages her own anxiety and gladly shares her success strategies in heartfelt public speaking. Elke's focus is on building people's strengths.

Frame of Reference

- ✧ Curiosity
- ✧ Mystery
- ✧ Discovery
- ✧ Guidance
- ✧ Leadership
- ✧ Non-positional, flexible, client-centred solutions

Elke's Own Creative Daily Principles and Practices

+ Daily gratitude journaling, morning and evening.

+ Long meditative walks through nature.

+ Writing poetry.

+ Community drumming workshops.

+ Learning to play the flute and the piano.

+ Hiking, mountain biking, kayaking, and sketching in the great, wondrous outdoors.

+ Inspirational reading.

+ Exploring philosophy and spirituality.

+ Exploring life, love, and the universe.

+ Expressing it all in painting and sketches.

Please write to the publisher to let Elke know how this book works for you, or what you would like to see added to future editions.

The Artist's Reply

1060 Partridge Lane, Bracebridge, ON P1L 1W8
Tel: 705-646-2300
Email: elkescholz@theartistsreply.com

Visit www.elkescholz.com:
Free downloads, posters, radio talks, YouTube videos,
and many more resources.

To book Elke for speaking engagements and workshops:
Tel: 705.646.2300
Email: elkescholz@theartistsreply.com

Available in print and ebook format online or inquire at your local bookstore

ORDER MORE COPIES

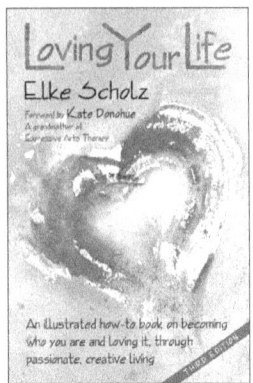

**Loving Your Life,
³rd edition**

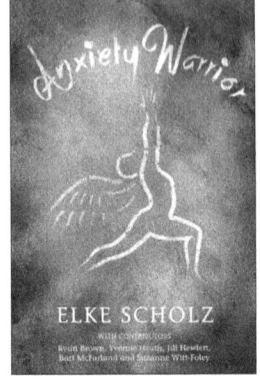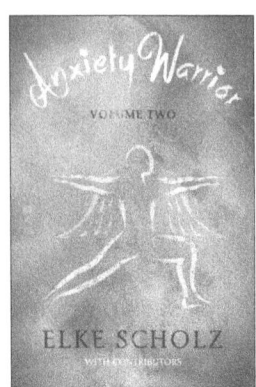

**Anxiety Warrior,
Volumes One and Two**

The third addition of this award-winning book with a foreword by Kate Donohue, a grandmother of EXA. Explore your creative mindfulness in this expressive arts book. Use it for daily inspirations, creative exercises and practices, for personal use, and in workshops. It is a fun and refreshing practical approach for well-being and for coming back to who you are.

Anxiety Warrior Volume One *came from seeing so many people in my private practice looking for strategies to lower anxiety. After many public talks, the need to make these strategies accessible became evident. Along with myself, there are five contributors — all professionals who are passionate about their work and empowering people.*

Anxiety Warrior Volume Two has delved deeper into more resources, and shares heart-felt, heroic stories of people like us.

The two volumes together make a very complete resource for managing and lowering anxiety. Each has a rich uniqueness in its offering.

Also available from The Artist's Reply

1060 Partridge Lane, Bracebridge, ON P1L 1W8
Tel: 705-646-2300   elkescholz@theartistsreply.com

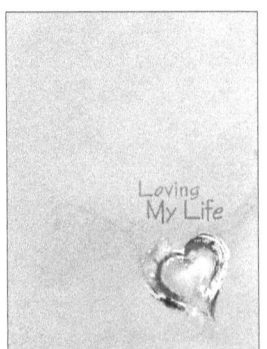

"Loving My Life" Journal

Journaling is a valuable activity that changes the neural pathways in our brain. Writing "it" down is a way to lessening our burdens. There is much research backing up the benefits of journaling. This journal provides [27] *ideas to help initiate some personal exploration. Try, explore and play. Discover the ones you like and the ones that give you the most energy.*

www.ingramcontent.com/pod-product-compliance
Lightning Source LLC
Chambersburg PA
CBHW070905120626
46546CB00001B/147